The Tib[...]
of Good [...]

The Hidden Treasure of the Turquoise Way

The Preliminary Practice of Yuthok Nyingthig Ngöndro

A Spiritual Practice of Traditional Tibetan Medicine

Dr. Nida Chenagtsang

Sorig Publications

Reprinted by Sorig Press UK 2013

Contents

PART 3   THE APPLICATION

The Tibetan Art of Good Karma

The Yuthok Nyingthig is an essential practice for everyone. It takes you on a journey where you'll come face to face with the ancient world of Tibetan medicine and shows how we can better approach and deal with every facet of life.

Drawing on the lineage of various masters lead by the ultimate heart of Yuthok himself, Dr Nida presents a series of practices to help us explore our connection to all phenomena and live with conscious thought, "the finest art of good karma is to live with awareness."

The genius of Yuthok was such that he produced an effective yet straightforward spiritual practice, so that doctors or those in healing professions could connect with him and develop truly great skills.

Whether you have an interest in Tibetan Medicine, Buddhism or simply to live a good life, the Yuthok Nyingthig delivers a simple yet sacred practice that, with guidance, offers immense benefit achievable in 7 days.

Dr Nida Chenagtsang is a Tibetan born medical doctor trained in the ancient teaching of Traditional Tibetan Medicine. He is the Director of the International Academy for Traditional Tibetan Medicine (IATTM) and the Co-Founder of the International Ngak Mang Institute (NMI), established to preserve and maintain the Rebkong Ngakpa culture within modern Tibetan society. He has published several books and articles on TTM and travels the globe actively teaching and treating patients.

Preface

The original text for this book was written in English by Dr Nida Chenagtsang under the title of 'The Art of Good Karma'.

Later in 2009 it was published in Italian (L'Arte del Buon Karma) and subsequently in 2010 in Portuguese (A Arte do Bom Karma).

With Dr Nida's permission, the original English version has been re-edited and renamed to this present artefact 'The Tibetan Art of Good Karma'.

This publication is the first title in English for Sorig Publications, a publishing house specifically developed under the guidance of Dr Nida for the purpose of producing and distributing texts on topics related to Traditional Tibetan Medicine and healing arts.

Throughout the entire process of this publication, many people have been instrumental in their support, emotionally, financially and demonstratively by assisting with review, suggestions, logo design, cover design etc. Thanks to Alessandro Petrini for the creation of the book cover, the Sorig Publication logo and for his support in text and photos. Special thanks to Rae Saleeba, Jenny McAuliffe and Virginia De Santis for their wisdom.

Naturally this book could not exist without the very person who gave it birth, Dr Nida Chenagtsang. All credit for this book is entirely reserved for Dr Nida.

Any errors or omissions in this re-edited version of the English edition fall chiefly with the editor.

Gabriella Sanelli
Editor, Sorig Publications

Foreword

The Yuthok Nyingthig practice is the secret path of Tibetan physicians, yogis and healers. It is an ancient tradition well suited to modern times primarily for the reason that the practice is very short and effective. It gives a deep spiritual understanding and infinite healing power, as well as a most secret spiritual realisation.

Dr Nida Chenagtsang is a certified Traditional Tibetan Medical doctor, who has completed training and practice of both the Four Medical Tantra and the Yuthok Nyingthig. I'm glad that he is bringing the authentic Tibetan medicine and Yuthok Nyingthig teachings to the world. By doing this, he is making a great contribution to both the preservation and development of Tibetan medicine in the 21st century.

Tibetan medicine focuses on the prevention and cure of all kinds of disease. This natural medical science deals with those individuals who are in need. Equally, the Yuthok Nyingthig is for universal healing for all sentient beings. This union of medicine and spiritual elements are essential to the Tibetan tradition and is referred to as *Mencho Zungdrel* i.e. the combination of Medicine and Buddha Dharma.

My wish is that this book will benefit many people, and may Yuthok bless them with his ultimate compassion and love.

I pray to Medicine Buddha and Yuthok to protect and support Dr Nida's work and may all his wishes be fulfilled.

Professor Dr Gojo Wangdui
Tibetan Medicine University
Lhasa, Tibet, 2009

Traditional Tibetan Medicine

Sowa Rigpa is Tibetan for Traditional Tibetan Medicine (TTM). It is the natural medical science of Tibet and is metaphorically compared to a large garden; an introduction is usually represented using the image of three trees.

In Traditional Tibetan Medicine, herbs, plants and trees play an important role. The main concept is that a healthy tree is like a healthy human being; a tree needs clean air, fresh water, adequate light and space in order to stay healthy and the same principle also applies to humans, every person needs the same elements in order to keep his/her health in balance.

Many of the principles and concepts in the Tibetan culture and its ancient medical system are originally based on the study of nature, trees, plants and the behaviour of wild animals. The results of these observations and the derived concepts are then compared with human beings in general and their health. This knowledge can be applied to topics such as how balance of health is found, what types of energies affect it and how a person should live to retain good health.

As Tibetan medicine is a natural system based on the observation of nature, the study of Tibetan medicine is consequently simplified using natural elements such as the symbology of trees. This illustrates an ancient form of study in which the tree not only represents the human form but also serves as an intellectual guide for the medical teachings. The trees become a 'mind map' of all the aspects of Tibetan medicine.

It's worth noting that traditionally, the conventional and complete study of Tibetan medicine covers no less than ninety-nine 'trees of knowledge'. The ninety-nine trees are studied sequentially and it usually takes twelve years to study the complete system of Traditional Tibetan Medicine, with all its theoretical principles and practical exercises. In contrast however, more modern educational systems such as those employed in India and Tibet where the emphasis is on the theoretical part, it generally only takes five years.

For Mantra Healing, which is part of Traditional Tibetan Medicine, only the first three trees of the entire ninety-nine are relevant.

The State of Balance

The first tree describes the general condition or state of a person and it has two trunks.

It represents a healthy person in which body, energy and mind are in a state of balance. A human being generally needs balance in his/her energies; energy builds the connection between body and mind. If the energy becomes imbalanced then the body and mind also become imbalanced consequently resulting in illness. On the other hand, good balance results in a healthy body, a large amount of vital energy as well as a clear, stable and happy mind.

The term *energy* in this context refers to a dynamic power, considered to be the source of all existence. In the body it is the psychophysical principle of vital energy. This energy arises from the five elements: space, wind, fire, water and earth. In the Tibetan view these elements are sometimes considered to be five in number and at other times four. Sometimes the element of space is not counted because it is the form in which the other four elements are found i.e. without space, earth, water, fire and air cannot exist.

The quality of space is the emptiness and the potentiality in which all phenomena originate. Wind has the quality of movement, growth and development. Fire represents speed and heat which leads in turn to maturation. Water has the character of flow and cohesion and earth represents consistency and stability.

These four elements can then be divided into three qualities or energies. The first energy is wind, derived from the Wind element (*rLung*); the second energy is Bile (*mKhrispa*), derived from the fire element; the third energy is Phlegm (*Bad-kan*), which is derived from water and earth elements. These three qualities can be further divided into two natures or characteristics. Wind and phlegm are cold whereas bile is hot.

These three qualities, derived from the five/four elements, are known as humours or inner energies and have different aspects which bring about different functions:

1. Wind (*rLung*): arises from the elements of space and wind:

- Is related to movement and activity
- Regulates thought and speech
- Controls the nervous system, breathing and excretion
- Areas relating to the wind element include the head, neck, shoulders, chest, heart, upper abdomen, elbows, large intestine, pelvic bone, wrists, lower abdomen, hips, knees and ankles.

2. Bile (*mKhrispa*): arises from fire:

    - Is related to heat
    - Regulates the body temperature
    - Bodily functions include digestion, absorption of nutrition, catabolic function, hunger and thirst, courage, motivation and visions.

3. Phlegm (*Bad-kan*): arises from earth and water:

    - Has a cold nature
    - Bodily functions include cohesion, fluid, structural binding of the body, bodily fluids, anabolic functions, sleep, patience and tolerance.

The Causes of Imbalance

Where the first trunk of the first tree represents a healthy condition, the analysis and balance of different energies, the second trunk describes the types and causes of imbalance.

All diseases are the effect of incorrect behaviours which is their karmic function; good karma brings perfect balance or health and bad karma generates imbalance or disease.

According to Traditional Tibetan Medicine, negative causes are divided into two categories: primary and secondary causes:

- Primary causes arise from negative and destructive emotional states or views such as anger, aggression, lust, unhealthy attachment (desire) and ignorance.
- Secondary causes are persistent and repetitive factors such as wrong nutrition and lifestyle, the time (seasonal causes) and provocations.

Let's look a little more closely to the secondary causes. Of the secondary type, the main cause of illness is incorrect food and lifestyle. Consider the cause of death related to cardiovascular diseases, the main cause of this disease tends to lie in nutrition and lifestyle factors. Becoming aware of one's food and lifestyle and making adjustments to them can lead to a healthy state of being; factors can include aspects such as amount and quality of sleep, daily routine, eating times, work, rest, etc.

According to the Buddhist tradition "liberation lies in one's own hand" and Traditional Tibetan Medicine adopts the same approach with regard to health; it lies in one's own hand. So by analysing the cause of illness and taking action on the causes of imbalance, you can return to the first trunk which is a state of balance - balance in body, energy and mind.

Another secondary cause is time which relates to rhythms and fluctuations in the environment, the condition of light, the climate and its influence on humans. There are certain combinations of elements in each season which in turn are reflected in bodily energies, dietary customs and behaviour.

The third secondary cause is provocation. Traditionally, provocation means that invisible spirits send negative energies to influence people and cause illness. The main view of provocation is that invisible beings inhabit the environment and influence the human world. This concept refers to the relationship of man within his natural environment. When we do not have a good relationship with our environment and the animals or when we destroy nature, we create something negative. An example of this is the pollution of air and water such as oil spills in the oceans and excessive carbon emissions, which consequently cause many health problems. It is believed that nature is the realm of the spirits, so it's important to cultivate a harmonious and respectful relationship with nature.

Methods of Diagnosis

The second tree is the tree of diagnosis and it has three trunks.

1. Inspection - the observation

   The patient's behaviour and appearance is closely examined; the first diagnosis is made by the analysis of urine, looking at aspects of colour, steam, bubbles, smell, sediments and oiliness, etc.

2. Palpation - the touch diagnosis

   Different aspects of the patient's pulse are palpated and two main aspects are differentiated; palpation for typological disposition and palpation for determination of pathological state. Tibetan doctors are trained in a special Tibetan style of pulse reading called *rtsapra* and they're also trained in chanting special mantras to increase their pulse reading power. This method is not mentioned in the *rGyud-bZhi* but only in the Yuthok Nyingthig and is considered a secret practice.

3. Anamnesis - the case history

   The patient is asked about lifestyle, diet, sensations, emotional and physical states, etc.

Healing Methods

The third tree is the tree of treatment and in Traditional Tibetan Medicine, methods of treatment generally falls into four basic categories:

1. Therapeutic Diet - the best treatment method

2. Modifications to lifestyle factors - daily routine, times of sleep, likes and dislikes, etc

3. Medication - Tibetan pharmacology uses herbs, minerals and small amounts of substances from animals

4. Application of External Therapies - Primary therapies are massage, acupuncture, moxibustion and cupping. Secondary forms of therapy include herbal baths, blood-letting, compresses, stick therapy and Mongolian Moxibustion.

According to the *gter-ma* tradition, Mantra Healing is the fifth trunk. Mantra Healing can be used separately as a treatment in its own right, or it can be combined with any of the four above mentioned treatment modalities in order to enhance their effects. When used in conjunction with diet, mantras can be used to empower foods for therapeutic purposes or to detoxify contaminated foods. Around the home, mantras may be used to create a more comfortable living space or to enhance communication and increase productivity in the work environment. Written mantras can be worn as amulets in order to protect from accidents, injury or to ward off spirit provocations.

Mantras can be combined with herbal medications to enhance their effects. During the compounding of Traditional Tibetan medicines many healing mantras are recited, incorporating the energy of sound into these complex combinations of herbs and minerals. We're able to use mantras in conjunction with Traditional Tibetan external therapies such as Ku Nye *(bsKu mNye)* massage, acupuncture, moxibustion, cupping and laying-on of heated stones or herbal compresses.

In summary, the general aims of Traditional Tibetan Medicine can be explained in two parts.

1. Preventive aspects

   Prevention of illness through correct lifestyle and diet are fundamental to Traditional Tibetan Medicine. In this modern age, most chronic diseases arise as a result of imbalance of mental attitude, incorrect lifestyle and incorrect diet. Diabetes and cardiovascular disease are well-known examples of this.

2. Curative aspects

Once imbalance arises, overt disease become manifest and it is then necessary to re-create balance through working on the underlying causes and effects. This means, in the first instance, attending to dietary and lifestyle factors, and then making use of herbal therapies and external therapies.

The Philosophy of Space and Time

The most important philosophical base for Traditional Tibetan Medicine is the interdependent origination of phenomena, which in Tibetan language is called *tendrel*. This philosophical view is accurately represented in Tibetan; *ten* means interdependent and *drel* means interconnection. The teachings essentially illustrate that nothing can exist by itself, everything is interconnected and co-existing. Our body, energy and mind are perfectly interdependent with the environment and with nature, co-existing with every single small object that is part of the greater universe. Everything is linked both directly and indirectly through visible and invisible energy, where great space and time are one in their primordial state.

The Sanskrit word *shunyata* is one of the most important terms in Mahayana Buddhism. It is composed of *shunya* which means empty, open, unsubstantial or nothing, and the substantive suffix *ta*. *Shunyata* is therefore the emptiness, openness, the non-substantiality of phenomena. However it does not mean a vacuum or nothingness. One may ask emptiness of what? It is in fact the emptiness of terms, mental constructions and projections. Emptiness is only that which is free of terms, categories, values, etc.

Opposed to the term emptiness is the term substantiality or inherent self existence. The expression below demonstrates the tendency in which phenomena are present in words or qualities.

All that which is 'A' can not be 'not-A'. When a thing is attributed as 'A', then a separation takes place between the things 'A' and the things 'not-A'

According to Buddhist philosophy, the confusion in this concept is that neither of the things *own* such attributes, nor do they *exist* in such a distinguished way.

The lack of inherent self-existence means that nothing comes into existence on its own and that nothing is unvarying in its appearance and substance.

The description of a tree can serve as an example. It is made of numerous cells from which some create the bark, others the wood and still some others the roots and leaves. If a leaf falls from a tree, then we consider the cells that, until that point we regarded as part of the tree, to now be separate from the tree and now an individual leaf. However it falls onto the ground where it will rot among other leaves, subsequently becoming nutrient for the tree and other leaves.

If our eyes were open to see subtle interdependence, we would then see an uninterrupted exchange of gas and substance with the atmosphere of the earth and countless organisms. We refer to it simply as a tree, but in reality we're dealing with an extremely complex phenomenon that is in a constant state of movement and exchange. If only a single factor is removed from the chain, leading to the appearance of the phenomenon, then the phenomenon disappears. Then it would be without a self i.e. with non-inherent verbal or conceptual attributions. Each phenomenon or object can be analysed in this way.

The Buddhist concepts 'emptiness of inherent self-existence', 'non-duality' and 'inseparability' are expressions for the alternating connection of all phenomena in an all-embracing, undivided and inseparable causal/conditional net. All beings, including human beings, are part of this net. As human beings we find ourselves continually exchanging and moving. We come to being through the substances of our parents, we are born, we breathe, we eat, we need movement, light and a certain temperature, etc. Nevertheless, during our life our cells continually die and new ones are created so that every seven years, we are in fact a completely new person. Everything is dependent on many factors and everything is movement, space and time, having never been created and never destroyed.

"Emptiness is form and form is emptiness" - Buddha

The nature of all existence is emptiness, and emptiness manifests within all existence, so emptiness is the form or wholeness, and there is no separation between existence and non-existence. Space and time arise or manifest through emptiness and that which is perfectly created by a clear and omni-pervasive mind. Once one realises the nature of mind, there is no longer any distinction made between subject and object, as reflected in Yuthok's song:

"In the clarity and emptiness of my mind,
the ineffable authentic state,

Bliss is omni pervasive, arising unceasingly and,

Emptiness and compassion are undifferentiated.

Hence, the phenomena created by mind are naturally liberated."

THE TRADITION OF
YUTHOK NYINGTHIG NGÖNDRO

A Spiritual Practice

The Yuthok Nyingthig (*gYu Thog sNying Thig*) is the most important and unique spiritual practice for Traditional Tibetan Medicine doctors, astrologers and healing practitioners, as well as for lay men and women.

It is a Tibetan medicine spiritual practice. *Nyingthig* is a common word in Tibetan Buddhist Schools and a few texts make reference to *Nyingthig*. For example, the *Longchen Nyingthig*, a spiritual practice taught by Longchen Rabjampa (1308—1369) and the *Karma Nyingthig*, the teachings of Karma Rangchung Dorje (1284—1339) who was the third great Karmapa.

Nying means heart and *Thig* means the essential, so a more complete meaning is 'Yuthok's essential heart teaching' or 'The Innermost Essence of the Teaching of Yuthok'.

The practice was composed with the intention of leading practitioners to experience the union of medicine with spiritual practice. This awareness is realised through the harmonious integration of body, mind and energy in the subtlest form of the five elements.

The series of teachings presented in this book are based on the Yuthok Nyingthig Original Text and Commentaries. The original Tibetan text is called **Yuthok Nyingthig Ladrub Dugngal Munpa Selvai Nyimi Odser** (*gYu Thog sNying Thig bLa sGrub sDug bsNgal Mun Sel nyi ma'i od zer*) which means 'The Innermost Essence of the Teaching of Yuthok, Guru Practice - the sun light that eliminates the darkness of suffering'.

The Yuthok Nyingthig is a Buddhist styled spiritual practice which brings harmony and peace for both self and others. It's not only a life philosophy and a great living art, it's also a great secret path to realising *Rainbow Body* which is the dissolution of the physical body into the essence of the five elements, disappearing into a 'body of light', typically leaving behind only fragments of hair and finger nails. Rainbow Body (*'ja lus*) or light body (*od sku*) is the highest spiritual realisation in the Tibetan spiritual tradition.

Historical Background

Originally the Yuthok Nyingthig was a secret spiritual practice of the Yuthok family and only ever transmitted through direct family lineage. In the eighth century, the elder Yuthok received many Vajrayana teachings including Mahamudra and Dzogchen (*rDzogschen*); however his main practice was the family's own secret practice. Through this he and his wife achieved *Rainbow Body*. At that time it was called the Dudtsi Mendrub (*bDud rTsi sMan sGrub*), the 'Nectar Medicine Practice' and became known as the 'Yuthok Family Nectar Medicine'. It was only practiced by their family and passed down many generations for centuries.

In the twelfth century, the young Yuthok Yonten Gonpo (1126—1202).was transmitted the teaching by his father

Yuthok also received this teaching from Khadroma Palden Tringva (*mkha'groma dpalldan phrengba*), the Medicine Dakini of Glorious Chain. Through visions, she gave permission that this secret teaching was at first to be transmitted to only one very close disciple, who then could transmit it to many qualified Doctors in the future. From then the teachings became known as the Yuthok Nyingthig.

As a result of practicing this teaching, the younger Yuthok and his wife also achieved *Rainbow Body*; their body, energy and mind dissolved back to the primordial state of the five elements.

It is said that Yuthok Yonten Gonpo the younger created two jewels; the Four Medical Tantras (*rGyud-bZhi*) and the Yuthok Nyingthig (*gYu Thog sNying Thig*). He gave the teachings and transmission of both jewels to his heart-disciple Sumtöng Yeshé Zung (*Sum sTon Yeshes gZhugs*) who maintained and perpetuated this tandem lineage of the Four Medical Tantras and the Yuthok Nyingthig.

The Yuthok Nyingthig is a secret teaching for those who wish not only physical and mental health but also to achieve absolute spiritual progress. Through this great path, Sumtöng realised perfect spiritual liberation.

Yuthok prophesied that in the future many Tibetan medicine doctors and healers would benefit from this practice.

Direct Lineage

As mentioned, the earliest Yuthok Nyingthig tradition was the Yuthok family spiritual practice, up until the twelfth century, when Yuthok the Younger transmitted it to Sumtöng Yeshé Zung, the first non-familial lineage holder of the Yuthok Nyingthig and the Four Medical Tantra.

Sumtöng in turn transmitted the Yuthok Nyingthig to his heart disciple Yeshe Shonnu. Then, in accordance with Yuthok's prophecy, the Yuthok Nyingthig teachings were transmitted to all people who wished to receive them. Ultimately, many people received and practiced this teaching and achieved the highest result.

In the fourteenth century, Zurkhar Nyamnyid Dorje (AD 1439—1476) had visions of Yuthok asking him to review and re-edit the Four Medical Tantra and Yuthok Nyingthig because some practitioners were not practicing in the correct way and the teachings needed to be clarified.

So Zurkhar re-edited the Yuthok Nyingthig and added one chapter about medical treatment. When he completed the addition, he subsequently taught it to many students and founded the Zurlug tradition of Tibetan medicine, the Zur School. It became one of the two largest schools of Tibetan medicine in history. Through Zurkhar's disciples, the Yuthok Nyingthig and the Four Medical Tantra teachings spread and developed all over Tibet.

In the seventeenth century, the Yuthok Nyingthig was the main spiritual practice of the Chagpori Tibetan Medical College which was the place where the original text was first published. The Chagpori students had to study the Four Medical Tantra and its Commentaries, Astrology and Philosophy however their main spiritual practice was the Yuthok Nyingthig which they practiced every day. It was the first time that the Yuthok Nyingthig was practiced in a large group in a medical college.

Over time, the many highly qualified Chagpori Medical doctors were invited to places all over Tibet, parts of Mongolia and China and consequently carried their medical tradition of the Four Medical Tantra and the Yuthok Nyingthig spiritual practice everywhere. Thus, as Yuthok had wished, his 'Two Jewels' were finally globally established. Since that time, the teachings have always been transmitted through highly qualified doctors and the authentic golden lineage is still unbroken today.

Lhasa Mentsi Khang (sMan-rTsis Khang) also practiced the Yuthok Nyingthig as the basis of their spiritual path right up until the Chinese communist invasion of Tibet. During the Cultural Revolution, many Doctors maintained their practice secretly; their efforts ensured that to this day, the Yuthok Nyingthig lineage has never been broken.

Khenpo Troru Tsenam was the greatest Tibetan medicine doctor of our time. He was not only the main lineage holder of the Troru Kyagyud tradition; he was also highly qualified in Nyingma study and practices. He was the most respected Tibetan scholar and doctor of the twentieth century and taught the Four Medical Tantra many times in Lhasa and other areas of Tibet. As the main lineage holder of Yuthok Nyingthig, he transmitted the teaching to his close disciples and it's thanks to his immense compassion and wisdom that Yuthok's main teachings, the Four Medical Tantra and Yuthok Nyingthig, are once again strongly flourishing after the Cultural Revolution.

One of his main disciples Khenpo Tsultrim Gyaltsen was a great Buddhist scholar, philosopher, astrologer and doctor. He had received the Yuthok Nyingthig from a few different Tibetan masters but he received the main essential teaching from Khenpo Troru Tsenam after which he transmitted the teachings to his closest disciples in Lhasa.

I have been fortunate to receive the complete Yuthok Nyingthig teachings from both Khenpo Truro Tsenam and Khenpo Tsultrim Gyaltsen. By applying careful study and practice I was able to have many of my doubts clarified by my precious medicine gurus and, under their guidance, Guru Yoga became a sacred and unique spiritual practice in my life. From 1989 to 1998, I completed my Four Medical Tantra study and practice in Amdo, Lhasa, and other parts of Tibet. The unbroken lineage has been transmitted by both Khenpo Truro Tsenam and Khenpo Tsultrim Gyaltsen to many doctors. Khenpo Tsultrim Gyaltsen would say that if you are unable to perform or follow all of the various practices, you can just do the Yuthok Nyingthig. It is a very practical and simple practice yet it is a complete and definite path to spiritual enlightenment.

Micho Khedrub Gyatso Rinpoche (*Alag Jamyang*) is the most well known and most respected lineage holder of the Yuthok Nyingthig practice and Tibetan medicine in the Amdo region of Tibet. He received the Yuthok Nyingthig teachings from Khenpo Truro Tsenam and today, Alag Jamyang is the holder of the Yuthok Nyingthig lineage in Tibet. He ensures that the Yuthok Nyingthig tradition continues to grow everywhere and through him, we're able to spread Yuthok's blessing to the many that are in need. He has granted permission for me to transmit this teaching further.

A Non-Sectarian Tradition

The Yuthok Nyingthig teaching is based on Vajrayana or Tantric system of Tibetan Buddhism. Although it mainly belongs to the Nyingma or old school of Tibetan Buddhism, Yuthok taught it to people who are involved in medicine and other healing practices as well as those who felt a close connection to him.

Yuthok Nyingthig is not a sectarian tradition; historically the practice can be found in all the schools of Tibetan Buddhism. The Yuthok Nyingthig is practiced by all Tibetan Buddhist schools however it is mainly studied and practiced by Tibetan doctors and healers.

In the Nyingma School, many people practiced the Yuthok Nyingthig because Yuthok himself was a Ngakpa and belonged to the Nyingma school. Many scholars and masters consider that the Yuthok Nyingthig is of the Terma (*gter-ma*) tradition which is most strongly connected to the Nyingma School. The largest collection of Terma, the Rinchen Terzod (*rin* chen *gter mdzod*) 'The Great Treasury of Precious Termas' was from the nineteenth century and it contained a short version of the Yuthok Nyingthig practice.

In the Kagyu and Sakya Schools we also find Yuthok Nyingthig practitioners especially those involved in Tibetan medicine. Many Geluk monasteries such as Labrang and Kumbum have medical colleges and all medical colleges practice the Yuthok Nyingthig as their main professional spiritual practice.

Yuthok Nyingthig may be a non-sectarian tradition but it has its own characteristics and style so it's important to gain a clear understanding of it and not dilute or infuse it with other practices. Other teachings require their own style of Ngöndro practice according to their tradition and it is important to respect every tradition by making a choice and maintaining a clear and simple way for a particular spiritual practice.

Some people complete the Yuthok Nyingthig Ngöndro and then think they have finished a Tibetan Buddhist Ngöndro, believing that they can now go on to receive all other teachings from other traditions. This is not the right way of thinking and can create confusion. It is extremely important to realise that when you have finished the Yuthok Nyingthig Ngöndro, it is essentially the base practice of the Yuthok Nyingthig path and not for any other teaching. Other traditions have their own paths.

In some cases people may have completed other practices and would now like do the Yuthok Nyingthig practice as well so as to make a connection with Yuthok or to receive his blessings. This concept is quite common. You can do the seven days of Yuthok Nyingthig practice and then continue your other practices afterward. Other practices can take many weeks or months to complete and some people are disappointed that they're not able to complete other types of Ngöndro as quickly as the Yuthok Nyingthig. By completing the seven days practice of the Yuthok Nyingthig Ngöndro, you're in a position to feel happy and fulfilled that you've done a complete practice in a short space of time.

For the Yuthok practice, there is no obligation to do it every day. Once you finish the seven days of the retreat, you can practice when you have time. As Yuthok promised, invoking him for just one second is the same as praying to other gurus for a month. If we believe in Yuthok's practice we must trust Yuthok's words; if we trust his word and we do his practice whenever we can, his extraordinary immediate blessing power is always present with us.

If you enjoy this practice, you should consider repeating it seasonally or yearly. For myself, I have done that and found that each time I do the practice, my foundation improves and is always stronger and more stable.

The Four Medical Tantra says "If there is no spiritual (Buddha Dharma) practice, then there is no real happiness in life." For this reason, it's important that physicians or healers have a spiritual practice and the Yuthok Nyingthig is specifically that, a path to spiritual development to achieve balance.

Traditional Tibetan Medicine is known as the 'Wise Man's Medicine' (*Drangsrong Lugs*) and has a close relationship with Tibetan Buddhism, but is not a Buddhist medicine. Tibetan medicine is a natural herbal medical system and for everyone, not for only one group of people or one nation; natural medicine is beyond cultural and political limitations.

In the past, there were some misunderstandings about Tibetan medicine because much of the study and practice of Tibetan medicine and of the Medicine Buddha was taught in monasteries so it was assumed that Tibetan medicine was strictly a Buddhist medicine. The reality is that Tibetan medicine is not a Buddhist medicine and in the Root Medical Tantra's first chapter, it makes reference to "This is the Wise Man's Medicine". If it was only a Buddhist medicine then the Medicine Buddha may have said, "This is Buddhist Medicine". By referring to it as the "Wise Man's Medicine" it gives an indication of its true purpose; that Traditional Tibetan Medicine is the perfect natural medicine for everybody without exception.

In Traditional Tibetan Medicine, the Medicine Buddha is the embodiment of health or balance for humankind, representing the possibility to achieve Buddhahood and eliminate the primary causes of all imbalances. The lapis lazuli Buddha represents space and at the same time, he is the essence of the absolute and true nature of our mind.

The relationship between Tibetan medicine and Tibetan Buddhism is such that they support each other. Tibetan medicine uses Buddhist philosophies such as the three mental poisons as the primary cause of illness, the theory of interdependence and a Buddhist style of healing. Tibetan Buddhism uses Tibetan medicine to learn more about health and curing people from the aspect of altruism; in the past most Tibetan physicians were Buddhist.

The great Yuthok also said that there is no single difference between the Four Medical Tantra and any other Tibetan Buddhist Vajrayana tantra. It is important to remember that the Four Medical Tantra is not just a medical text.

The Original Text

The Yuthok Nyingthig Original Text is an exposé of Yuthok's spiritual teachings. Yuthok considered spiritual practices, yoga and meditation to be an integral part of every physician's training. The original text contained:

1. The Ngöndro practice - The Preliminary Practice as the basic foundation

2. Four forms of Guru Yoga with Yuthok

    i. Outer Guru Yoga - this focuses on Yuthok with the Four Medicine Dakinis and the Mantra of the entire Yuthok mandala, a seven day practice.

ii.   Inner Guru Yoga - this focuses on Yuthok in the form of the Medicine Buddha and includes the practice of the Five Buddhas and activating our five chakras, a seven day practice.

iii.   Secret Guru Yoga - a practice on three roots as Guru Yoga, a seven or more day practice.

iv.   Union Guru Yoga - a daily life practice of Yuthok Guru Yoga with a short mantra.

3. A major chapter on Tibetan Medical Yantra (*'khrul 'khor*) Yoga. There are about eighteen movements providing the base for balance, health and path to spiritual enlightenment.

4. Fifteen chapters on the study of Physical Medicine and Pathology such as disturbances of the three humours, infectious diseases, pain, trauma, poisons, causes of disease, their symptoms and how to treat them through diet, life style, medicine and external therapies.

5. A complete set of Vajrayana practices:

i.   Khyed Rim (*bsKyed Rim*) - A Generation or Creation practice, a practice of the three roots. This is in the form of Guru Yoga.

ii.   Dzog Rim (*rDzogs Rim*) - A Completion practice which contains information on the following Six Yogas:

• Tummo (*gtummo*) – The divine fire yoga practice which generates our inner fire element to eliminate the root of all imbalances and increase perfect bliss and wisdom.

• Gyulu (*sgyu lus*) – The illusory body practice, to discover and experience the real nature of our body and all existence.

• Bardo practice on death, the ways of total freedom after death and how to choose a good rebirth.

• Phowa (*'pho ba*) - A practice on how to die in peace and the final spiritual journey.

• Odsel (Od gSal) - Clear light yoga. This practice is to understand the true nature of our mind and awareness of presence.

• Milam (*Rmi lam*) - Dream yoga practice. This is for realising the hidden aspects of our mind and energy and how we can be free from all types of blockages and emotions.

iii. Dzogchen (*rDzogs chen*) - The Great Perfection practice or great ending practice. *Dzog* means end and *chen* means great so it means 'greatly ends the samsara'. This particular chapter of the text is referred to as 'The Self-Liberation of Samsara-Nirvana'. It is a secret path for realising the final Rainbow Body *('ja lus)* or light body *(od sku)*, through two main ways;

- First - to break through all logic and focus on four points: 1) None, emptiness, the nature of all phenomena is always in the state of emptiness, all beyond space and time, 2) One, single nature, in non-dualistic dimension, all in one and one in all, 3) Omnipresent, all pervasive, beyond mind and space and 4) Spontaneous manifestation, absolute self manifestation and perfect by itself.

- Second - the practice on the energies of lightness and darkness and accumulation of cosmic power to develop the divine light body or Rainbow Body.

iv. Mendrub (*sMan sGrub*) - Practices on healing and protection mantras, medicine rituals as well as practices for the medical protectors.

6. Instructions for a special form of pulse diagnosis where the practitioner must engage in spiritual retreat and specific practices for a month as preparation prior to reading a patient's pulse.

The Yuthok Nyingthig practice itself is associated with the development of special powers of omniscience and clairvoyance which then help the physician to become a greater physician or healer.

In the original text, there are explanations given for all of these practices as well as information on how to integrate them with the practice of medicine. This book will cover the first part, the Ngöndro practice which is the base or foundation of the Yuthok Nyingthig.

The meaning of Ngöndro

Ngöndro means preliminary practice or preparation. By using the term 'preliminary practice' it may seem to besomething very basic, and in some respects it is basic, but at the same time it is very important. We could call it a *basic essential practice*. We could compare it to the upbringing of a child; the family and early school education are both rudimentary yet important aspects for the child's development. In a similar way the Yuthok Nyingthig Ngöndro practice is extremely useful and essential for beginners to Buddhism.

If we imagine the building of a house, the foundations need to be very stable and strong. Likewise, if we want to develop our spiritual practice, we need our basic framework to be strong. Spiritual practice is like a building which can have one, two or more floors. Buddha mentioned there are ten levels or *bumis* and the higher our building or spiritual practice go, the stronger our foundation needs to be. By doing the Ngöndro we set up the foundation of our spiritual practice.

In the Buddhist tradition, Ngöndro practices are often very demanding and considerable time, effort and dedication is needed to accomplish them, for example at least 100,000 prostrations, recitations of refuge, bodhicitta etc need to be completed.

My first Buddhist master was the great nun, Ani Ngakwang Gyeltsen. At birth she was recognised as the reincarnation of Taglung Tse Rinpoche, a very important master. Ani trained with her master the most famous female practitioner Shugseb Jetsun Rinpoche (1865—1953) at Shugseb nunnery. After many years of practice she became highly qualified in *gtummo* yoga and Dzogchen practices. Her level of *gtummo* practice was so great that she spent most of her time outdoors or in high caves, frequently in extremely cold conditions. Her dreams were often omniscient and she helped many people in this way.

She was meditating in a cave when the Chinese arrested and imprisoned her. In one torture room the roof was made of ice. As she sat in her room, she practiced generating her *gtummo* heat so effectively that the whole ice roof collapsed. Once the police discovered her capacity they put water containers in her room at night to stop it freezing. They also tortured her by breaking her leg so she could not sit in a meditation pose. During her time in captivity, she spent much of her time weaving and whilst it appeared that she was simply keeping her hands busy, in reality she was effectively integrating everything she did and experienced into her practice.

Eventually, after many years Ani was released from prison and was invited to return to her nunnery. But instead of returning to the comfort of her nunnery, she instead decided to stay in Lhasa in her tiny room. All she had was her bed, a very simple kitchen and a shrine with a statue of her master, some dharma texts and nothing else. She spent all her time teaching individual students and on her own in meditation.

In 1991 I was very fortunate to meet her in Lhasa where she taught me the Longchen Nyingthig Ngöndro as a base spiritual practice. She advised me that it could take many years to complete this practice and that even in isolated retreat, it would still take almost six months.

While studying at the Tibetan Medical College in Lhasa, I finally completed my Longchen Nyingthig Ngöndro although it took me three years. Due to my studies I wasn't able to do six solid months of retreat; instead I practiced my Ngöndro in my dormitory every morning and evening sitting in my bed. I created a little retreat space by putting a curtain across the top of the bunk bed. My friends were very noisy and would talk loudly, drink alcohol and smoke which made it hard to keep focus, but that was only my karmic space. On many occasions I had to hide my altar as we were not permitted to use any Dharma items in the dormitory. My Longchen Nyingthig Ngondro practice was very challenging but once I start something, I always want to finish it. On a winter holiday from college, I travelled back home to Amdo and was able to practice my prostrations alone, it took more than forty days in a very strict retreat.

In the Tibetan culture if you say that you've completed a Ngöndro they assume that you've accomplished a really difficult practice, as though you've successfully passed an exam. As mentioned earlier, the reason we do Ngöndro with all its various repetitions is to build the foundation for our spiritual practice.

A number of people think that Ngöndro is very plain and simple and that it can never bring final spiritual realisation. In the modern western world it's common to hear people say that Ngöndro is not their style, it's only for beginners and not an important practice. Some people do Ngöndro in order to receive further teachings and practices as I did. My master advised me that I was only allowed to receive certain teachings after accomplishing the Ngöndro. I was young and really didn't think much of the meaning of the Ngöndro nor was I aware of its value; all I thought about was counting the number of prostrations and mantras, rushing to finish it as quickly as possible.

From my great root guru Chonyid Rinpoche, I received the complete Vajrayana teachings including the full steps of Dzogchen which I practiced as much as possible. During 1993 to 1998, I studied with Rinpoche in his place called Lamaling in Konpa and also in Lhasa. My guru taught that Ngöndro is very much the basis of all Vajrayana teachings however I was naive and thought Ngöndro is not that essential, it's a waste of time. A few years later, I learned about the importance of Ngöndro and I now wish to practice more and more Ngöndro. I would even venture to say it's the basis and heart of Tibetan Buddhism. Without the practice of Ngöndro and its understandings, we may never reach Buddhahood.

Tibetan history details that highly realised Buddhist masters would repeat a full Ngöndro each year. Their high level of realisation meant they were inherently aware of the importance of Ngöndro and for that reason would repeat it on a regular basis. One great and famous master Shardza Tashi Gyaltsen (1859—1935) who attained one of the last known occurrences of Rainbow Body was known for his yearly

Ngöndro practice. The great Lama Tsongkhapa (1357—1419) did so many prostrations that he left an imprint of his body on a stone. How amazing to think that one of the most highly qualified scholars did this simple practice so many times! The Ngöndro is a very demanding practice especially in our time poor modern society. It's often difficult to complete it in it's entirety in one go as people can rarely find six consecutive months to do the Ngöndro retreat. Our busy lifestyles can sometimes mean it takes so long to finish the practice that we end up doing it bit by bit or not in a correct way due to distractions.

Yuthok had foreseen the future where our busy times and distracting modern lifestyle would hinder our ability to practice the teachings. He prophesied that the Yuthok Nyingthig would be a suitable and convenient practice for us. In his prophecies, Yuthok made mention that in future times people (especially physicians and the like) would be too busy to dedicate a lot of their time to spiritual practice and for that reason, he reduced the practice to seven days. He decided to concentrate his energies, desires and accumulation of merits so that a person doing his practice could receive his blessings even in this time.

In the history of the Yuthok Nyingthig, Yuthok said:

"If a practice has no immediate blessing power, future people will desire a short practice as they won't have the effort for doing long practices, and they won't continue. Therefore if someone does my heart teaching for seven days without any distractions, they will be blessed.'

The Yuthok Nyingthig Ngöndro can be completed within seven days. Yuthok taught this spiritual practice in his own style, varying from other Ngöndro practices which consider a seven day Ngöndro practise as too short. Yuthok emphasised that doing this Ngöndro is equal to a traditional Ngöndro. Yuthok's main focus is that the Ngöndro practice should be put to good use, it's not just about counting recitations. It is with his blessing that seven days is sufficient to experience and understand the meaning of the Ngöndro following which we can incorporate it into our lives by helping patients and other people in need.

In Tibetan Buddhism there are many different Buddhas such as the Wisdom Buddha, Buddha of Compassion, Power Buddha, Medicine Buddha, Long life Buddha, Wealth Buddha etc. Why are there so many? Well, all of them have their own 'profession' and are specialists in their specific fields. Although they have the same underlying quality of Buddha, individually they demonstrate various different powers.

When it comes to the Medicine Buddha, he and Yuthok have energies that emphasise immediate blessing and ultimate healing. Because of Yuthok's merits, prayers and energy, even by performing a short day of this sacred practice, you will be immediately blessed. Unlike other traditions, where one has to accumulate huge numbers of actions, the Yuthok Nyingthig is exceptionally empowered with Yuthok's heart essence, guaranteeing your spiritual progress.

Historically, not everyone believed in Yuthok's teachings. One such man was a great master of Tibet who was called Karma Chagmed (1613—1678). He doubted Yuthok's theory that a short practice like that could achieve anything, so he decided to test it out. After only one week of retreat, Karma Chagmed wrote a short text about the Yuthok practice, suggesting to his disciples that they too should follow this practice, that the Yuthok Nyingthig practice could prolong life for everybody.

Some people might wonder that if the Yuthok Nyingthig practice is only for one week, then why are there many levels? It is a reasonable question. Firstly, it's very important to finish the Ngöndro practice followed by the first Guru Yoga of Yuthok. That in itself is already sufficient for those who desire only a short practice. Then, in the Outer Guru Yoga of Yuthok, there is the full mantra of Yuthok's mandala, for those who want to deepen their practice in a more profound way. Following that, they can continue on with the remaining levels, each level taking a week to complete.

Three Stages of Yuthok Ngöndro

Typically in other Ngöndro practices there are two different stages referred to as Common Ngöndro and Uncommon Ngöndro however the Yuthok Nyingthig Ngöndro has three main parts:

1.   Common Ngöndro (The Base)

     The base refers to the foundation of the Yuthok Nyingthig Ngöndro. The Common Ngöndro is simply for all common people so everyone is able to reflect on the meaning of life, to see the true nature of life. It has five important points and these can be practiced by thinking or meditating however if we're able to realise these through our own life experiences, it is even more effective.

     •   The difficulty in achieving a precious human life

     •   The impermanence of life

     •   The natural law of cause and effect.

- The consequence of living in Samsara, the worldly life

- The benefits of spiritual liberation

2.   Uncommon Ngöndro (The Path)

This is a special Buddhist concept which is different from our normal way of looking at our life. This is why it is known as the Uncommon practice. Dharma refers to the way or path, and everybody and every tradition has their own way of thinking and living according to it. Buddha's way of thinking is called Buddha Dharma and in this case, Buddha's style is called Uncommon to others. In the Yuthok Nyingthig tradition, there are seven aspects:

- Refuge

- Bodhicitta and the Four Immeasurables

- Prostration

- Mandala offering and Circumambulation

- Purification practice of Dorje Sempa

- Kusali practice

- Puja practice

3.   Routine Ngöndro (Karma Yoga)

Once we've completed the Uncommon Ngöndro we then need to establish a routine practice. Importantly this is something that can be practiced throughout our whole lives, whenever we can or when we desire to do something for the benefit of others, to help others and make others happy. We can achieve this through Karma Yoga.

In this way, daily life can be integrated into the practice ensuring mindfulness is part of everything we do. In the original text there are six important points:

- Be involved in charity projects especially those to help poor and sick people

- Find ways to save lives not just for your patients but for all people and animals. Always find ways to help others as much as possible

- Always strive to spread Yuthok's teachings especially the Four Medical Tantras and the Yuthok Nyingthig

- Create a clinic or a centre where those who are in need can receive help

- Make donations or offer your time to help build things that will benefit many beings such as community centres or animal shelters. Or participate in projects in poorer countries where they need things like wells and bridges.

- Liberate animals & protect the environment.

PART 1   THE BASE

The Common Ngöndro

A Precious Human Life

According to science the human body is the most complex and powerful machine in our world. In the Vajrayana tradition it is referred to as the Vajra body meaning the absolute body, one with no dualistic nature. In this view, both ancient wisdom such as Tibetan medicine and modern science agree that the human body is most precious and valuable.

Human life is the source of countless Buddhas and Bodhisattvas, it's a font of extraordinary energy and wisdom. We need to use this wisdom to be sure about the choices we make and use our knowledge and awareness to really analyse the paths that are open to us.

A human being is precious regardless of colour, culture, religion, nationality, gender, age or social circumstances. To enable us to fulfil our spiritual potential, good karma is needed to meet the many teachers and masters, to listen to their teachings. As important as these teachers are, we must still trust our own potential and intuition and take care not to follow dangerous paths that can lead us to faulty or improper spiritual traditions.

It's not so straightforward to have a balanced and healthy human body. It requires various suitable conditions such as healthy genes from our parents, proper lifestyle and diet, clean environment and surroundings, fresh water and food and so on.

For most of us, we're fortunate to have good health, food and shelter, a clean environment and we generally don't live in places of war, natural disasters or famine, or where people endure terrible hardship. Many of us have the ability and the free time to pursue spiritual matters. These conditions mean that we are experiencing a precious human re-birth; it would be a pity to not make the most of this situation. We are marvellous creations with limitless potential and we should not waste a single minute.

If you don't have much knowledge about your body, your vehicle for this life, you should take every opportunity to learn about it through both modern and traditional medicine for example anatomy, physiology and embryology. Today we are so fortunate that many great masters and teachings are easily available to us.

Meditation
At any time, take ten to twenty minutes to contemplate this precious human life. You can do this while walking, sitting or in even bed, just before falling asleep. Think of it as a meditation practice, it can be a very undemanding and simple way to focus your mind. Whenever possible, it is beneficial to talk about these things with your spiritual friends. At every opportunity, try not only to look for a clearer understanding but also to discover ways to be of benefit to others.

Once you begin to get a sense of the preciousness and bountiful potential of human life, you generate positive energy and you can transform it into a desire to help others. In that way, from this simple meditation, you can achieve something positive not only for yourself, but for others as well. It's important to value this precious human body, don't mistreat your own vehicle for enlightenment, think and act positively and both your body and mind will surely benefit. Even those with a physical disability can use their limitless potential of mind to benefit others.

The Impermanence of Life

"Life flickers in the flurries of a thousand ills,
More fragile than a bubble in a stream.
In sleep, each breath departs and is again drawn in;
How wondrous that we wake up living still!"

Nagarjuna

The nature of all phenomenona is impermanence, directly influenced by the natural cycle of cause and effect, the law of science. This means that everything is constantly changing in every instant.

As science now knows, the universe is always expanding, a perfect example of the state of impermanence. According to the Big Bang Theory in the creation of the universe, we're still riding the waves of that explosion as the universe continues to expand.

We are living in an impermanent space, with time constantly changing. From spring to summer, autumn to winter, the ever changing seasons are like a perfect guru, teaching us in the natural cycle of impermanence.

After billions of years, even the stars will one day become dust. Sometime ago, I conducted a class on Tibetan Medicine in Umbria, Italy. The students and I had the opportunity to visit a nearby astronomy station, where we had a chance to observe space and the stars. One of the guides showed us a star in the form of a cloud and said that this formation is actually the end of a star, a dying star. Seeing this offered me a deep understanding of the illusory and impermanent nature of the entire universe; every shooting star is our night guru, teaching us perfectly about impermanence.

Billions and billions of humans have lived and died on this planet and over 6 billion are living now, in another 100 years most of them will also be gone. They will be replaced by new generations again and again. Every one of those people was once just like us and one day, we will be like them.

Birth, life and death - none of us is beyond these realities. The wheel of life turns non-stop; all of us experience every year, every month, every day, every hour, every minute and every second. Billions of our cells are regenerating every second; even this body we know now is completely replaced every seven years.

The course of impermanence is like our first breath at birth or our first heart beat which started in the second month of gestation; since the first, they've never stopped. Similarly, each individual breath and heart beat manifests this state of impermanence as no two are ever the same. It's useful to be mindful of each breath and each heartbeat; our heart beats 100,000 times a day and every beat is a reminder of impermanence.

Sometimes we feel that time does not pass but in reality, time is constantly moving at high speeds, in fact most often we're so preoccupied in 'keeping time' that we don't notice how quickly time passes. Essentially, our life can be compared to only three days or ages; the day of studying (age 1 to 30), the day of working (age 30 to 60) and the day of medication (age 60 to 90), when we eventually depart to our final destination.

We all know when we were born but we can never know when we will die. After death, all is gone, so why do we struggle and fight for so much in this life? Looking back through history, we see so many terrible events have occurred due to some people's force of will or desire of power, yet in the reality of impermanence, their cause is pointless. After their death, their ego, emotions and power are all meaningless. So it's important that we think about our life carefully and do things that are helpful or useful for our family, society, people, animals and future generations and for our home planet.

Even in our own circle of friends and family, we can see how things continually change; the rich can become poor, the healthy people can become sick and friends can become enemies. Thus, everything we desire has the potential to become a cause for suffering.

From time to time when we notice a difference in our body such as wrinkles, grey hair or scars, we should not consider these as negative aspects of life but embrace them as an opportunity to accept and understand the nature of impermanence.

Even though everything is in a state of impermanence, it is important to keep a positive outlook; if people experience difficult periods such as panic attacks or depression, they should not take it too personally or severely. Both acute and chronic diseases may arise at any time where they can suddenly be taken ill or even disabled, so we should take every opportunity to practice and learn to maintain a clear perspective on the process of impermanence.

Meditation

Similar to the previous meditation practice, you should take ten to twenty minutes daily to think about the nature of impermanence and the cycle of life and death. You can do this whilst walking or sitting up in bed. Pay particular attention to your breath, knowing it is your life counter. Feel your pulse and become mindful of your heart beat, a reminder of your life and everything that beats in time and within every being.

Special note - People who have a tendency to suffer from panic attacks or depression should be careful with this meditative practice. Instead you should just count your breath, inhale for a count of four, hold for a count of three and breathe out for a count of five. Don't attempt to focus your mind on impermanence and death as it may lead to an increase in fear or anxiety in some people.

The main outcome of meditating on impermanence should be to inspire you to practice every day, to not waste a moment on superficial, pointless or harmful activities and to develop an awareness of the never ending cycle of life and death.

The Natural Law of Cause and Effect

The most natural cycle of cause and effect is called karma, which literally can be translated as 'action'. In Tibetan the word is 'Le Gyu Dre' *(las rgyu 'bras)*; *Le* means action, *Gyu* is cause and *Dre* is effect. This is the natural cycle of all phenomena; the energy of action creates a cause, and through action a cause makes an effect. If cause is without action then it can't create effect, therefore action is always the main process of karma.

There are two types of causes of karma; the first cause is the primary or primordial cause, it is un-changeable, and the second cause can be changed depending on how the action is processed. For example if we have a karmic seed we can affect that seed, it already exists but its future is up to us. If we plant it in good soil and give it clean air and water then the seed can grow and bear fruit. Therefore we can say that the seed is the first or primary cause and the action of planting and giving water is the secondary cause. If we alter this second aspect then we can change the plant's future. We should not think that karma is fixed or unchangeable, in reality karma is just up to us, every person has more than one potential future.

Karma does not only refer to your past lives. Many people find the idea of karma frightening or worrying, they think too much about

-36-

past negative actions. It is important to always strive for good karma here and now. In fact good karma is in your actions, it means to be honest, to have good intentions, tolerance, compassion and love and to keep in harmony with others. All that can bring a perfect future.

When we purify our past to keep a good present then there will be a better future; this is good karmic understanding and practice.

Every thought, each single action, every chance and opportunity is karma; and the finest art of good karma is to live with awareness.

Some people believe that living with awareness is likened to living in a special mental state which allows you to do anything you want no matter if it's good or bad. This is a dangerous misinterpretation and can be an assured path to the cause of negative karma. No matter what your state of mind, bad actions will bring a bad result.

Believing in Karma leads to good things:

- It helps you to accept things more easily
- It gives you a deeper understanding of self and others
- It opens the heart and naturally makes you a good person
- And it brings a peace and a better quality of life

Meditation
Take ten to twenty minutes to contemplate the natural cycle of cause & effect. You can do this at any moment, while walking, sitting or in even bed just before falling asleep. The result will be that you'll feel a deep desire to accumulate infinite good karma and merit throughout your entire life.

The Consequence of Living in Samsara

Of course human life is beautiful and full of hope, and it's the same for many animals as well. But through mindfulness and awareness we also see that this worldly life brings many consequences of pain and suffering, all at the high speed of Samsara.

Samsara means the wheel of the life, our worldly life in which the conflict and pain never ends. This is because we're not aware of the root cause of the suffering and pain in our lives.

What do we find in our lives nowadays? We find that many people suffer from poverty and hunger, others suffer from disease and pain, some suffer from war and natural disaster, and many people are mentally unhappy with common disturbances such as depression, anxiety, fear and panic. There is fighting between person to person, village to village, nation to nation and country to country, friendship and family conflicts, social problems, religion and political fights; there is much more suffering and conflict than there is happiness and harmony.

Once the wheel of Samsara has started it can't be easily stopped; birth, life, death, again and again the same cycle of birth, life and death continues - it's a wheel that turns on our suffering.

Meditation

Take ten to twenty minutes to reflect on Samara, the wheel of life. You can do this at any time, while walking, sitting or in bed. The result will be that you'll feel a real desire to find the perfect path to go beyond Samsara and dedicate time to your practice.

> *Special note* - People who have a tendency to suffer from panic attacks or depression should be careful with this meditation. You should instead just count your breath, inhale for a count of four, hold for a count of three and breathe out for a count of five. Don't attempt to focus your mind too much on the negativity of Samara as it may lead to an increase in fear or anxiety in some people.

The Benefits of Spiritual Liberation

Everything we desire has the potential to become a cause of suffering so it's important to discover a way to escape the endless cycle of Samsara.

Spiritual understanding is very effective when dealing with problems in our life and the path of the Buddha Dharma can help us to open our mind, to realise the meaning of life in a deep and profound way.

When we have an opened mind, there are fewer disturbances, we accept things more readily, we endure less troubles and conflicts and we're happier; essentially it can make us feel that life is good. Our practice helps to make our life easier, to have an opened mind and to accept things more easily and strive to be happier.

The three main points of Buddha Dharma are to:

- do virtuous things as much as possible
- avoid non-virtuous actions and
- tame ones own mind

Spiritual practice can be a preventative solution for mental disturbances and psychological problems. It can even lead to liberation from all suffering.

Meditation
Take ten to twenty minutes to reflect on Spiritual Liberation every day until you feel you have a deeper understanding of the benefits of Buddha Dharma. You can do this at any time. The result is that you're sure to experience a great practice and you'll never give up your spiritual path.

Summary of Common Ngöndro

Once you have studied and practiced these five points, you can then continue onto the Uncommon Ngöndro. It's essential however to always keep the five Common practices in your mind as they are the basis of your great spiritual journey.

PART 2   THE PATH

The Uncommon Ngöndro

Uncommon Ngöndro in Detail

Uncommon Ngöndro is a special Buddhist concept which is different from the normal way we think about our life. This is why it's called an uncommon practice or more precisely, an extraordinary practice. According to the Yuthok Nyingthig there are seven aspects to follow:

1) Refuge

2) Bodhicitta and the Four Immeasurables

3) Prostration

4) Mandala offering and Circumambulation

5) Purification practice of Dorje Sempa

6) Kusali practice

7) Puja practice

What is Meditation?

In Tibetan, the word for meditation is 'Gom' (bsGom) which originated from another word 'goms' (goms) meaning to become familiar with. It means to really know one's mind, energy and body. First we need to gain self-understanding and then expand that to a greater understanding of all existence. Yuthok often spoke of meditation in these terms. He said that it was not 'meditation', but becoming familiar, to completely understand, to have total awareness of the self.

There are many types of meditation. One type is called Gyergom (gyer bsgom) which means chanting meditation. This kind of meditation relates to the Nyingma tradition, the oldest Buddhist school. In this meditation style, the mind focuses on chanting words and their meaning, on being present and aware in every word. Your mind may have thoughts yet by maintaining awareness, you don't try to stop the thought, you simply let it pass in a balanced way. This process is easy for beginners.

Another common meditation is Shine (zhi gnas) where the focus is on calming the mind or relaxing the mind, keeping the mind in silence without motion. In this meditation, we stop our thoughts in order to achieve a non-moving state of mind. It can be difficult to achieve but once attained, all other meditations become easier. This is one of the foundation meditations to all other types of meditations.

Chegom meditation (*dpyad bsgom*) refers to an analytical meditation, to analyse philosophical views and to understand things by thinking. This meditation is very useful when you're unable to stop your mind from thinking. By using the mind in the correct way, by using the mind for meditation, one can prevent the mind from having many senseless thoughts.

In some kinds of meditation, we focus on our breath and this is known as Energy meditation. Through slow, gentle breathing we can control the mind. Once we can do this, the mind may not be easily distracted by anything, thus enabling us to be free from negative emotions and bad karma.

There are also movement meditations such as Walking meditation or Yoga movements which work on both body and mind. Through movement of the body, it makes it possible to work or calm the mind. As the body is more familiar than our mind, we can use the body as a gate to get inside the mind.

Mindfulness meditation is keeping your awareness on whatever you're doing i.e. allowing yourself to be in the present moment and not going over past memories or thinking about the future. For example when you brush you teeth or take a shower, we often allow the mind to think of a myriad of things rather than concentrating on what we're actually doing. Mindfulness meditation is about being in the moment, of not following thoughts and just keeping the mind in the here and now, with naked awareness. Doing anything with awareness whether it is standing, eating, talking or working, is all daily practice of mindfulness.

Each individual can have different meditation goals, one's capacity and wishes are often not aligned. In ancient times people practised meditation for higher goals, to reach spiritual enlightenment, however nowadays people seek out meditation for various reasons and with different motivations. Some people seek a calm and relaxed mind, rested body or to gain more energy. Others try it for healing or therapeutic benefits, there are those who wish to achieve magic powers or new experiences and of course, some are just following the new fashion.

The good news is that everyone can find their own ideal way of meditation. It's important to know that there are many types of meditations and each person can choose whichever style is most suitable for them. There is no one best practice for all people. It's just like food, every nation thinks their food is the best, we can't find a perfect food for all mankind.

The Buddhist style of meditation has one main goal; to achieve Buddhahood in order to help all sentient beings. Therefore additional less common meditation methods are needed.

In summary, there are three main different types of meditation:

- Body meditation - refers to the sitting position, walking, standing, yoga; all things which relate to using our body with awareness.
- Voice meditation - chanting mantra, singing prayers and songs; everything that connects with our voice through mindful activity.
- Mind meditation - calming the mind, resting the mind, analysing and thinking; everything which deals with the mind.

These three aspects can be done individually or combined together but at all times, it is important to develop your practice gradually.

Chanting in Sanskrit or Tibetan

Many spiritual traditions come from Asian countries where chanting is done in the original language. Some people think there is no real purpose to chant in the native language, that it's easier to chant in one's own language rather than the native tradition. But chanting in the original language has a number of real benefits which cannot be realised if chanting is done in a foreign way.

Mantras and sacred texts carry a vital energetic vibration which works through the sounds, not through the translation.

The original Sanskrit language was blessed by Buddha and other great Bodhisattvas. Likewise, the Tibetan language is empowered by many great practitioners and in both cases; there is a perfect energy within the native languages.

Learning a new language or chanting in a new language makes clever use of the brain which can bring about certain benefits to our health. We can maintain a healthy memory and active brain through learning new things and studying a new language is one of the best methods. Sometimes if we translate the native language, the translations may not be accurate and often dilute the original meaning. Learning a new vocabulary however allows you a deeper understanding.

Learning a new language can be difficult at first but like any good meditation practice, once it becomes familiar, everything is perfect. A good meditation practice helps you become more of a relaxed and uncomplicated person with infinite knowledge.

Refuge and Yuthok's Prayer

Taking Refuge in Yuthok—the Perfect Medicine Guru

རིགས་འདུས་བདེ་གཤེགས་རྡོ་རྗེ་འཆང་།།

Rig dü de sheg Dorje Chang
You who are the union of all sugatas and Vajradhara,

ཕྱོགས་དུས་དཀོན་མཆོག་གསུམ་གྱི་དངོས།།

Chog dü kön chog sum gi ngö
Essence of the Three jewels in the ten directions and three times,

བདག་གཞན་བྱང་ཆུབ་མ་ཐོབ་བར།།

Dak shen chang chub ma tob bar
Until I and all others achieve enlightenment,

སྙིང་ནས་དུས་ཀུན་གསོལ་བ་འདེབས།།

Nying ne nye war kyab su chi
From my inner heart I take refuge in you.

These four lines mean that we take refuge in Yuthok.

> (You are the) Union of all Buddhas and Vajradhara,
>
> Of the Three Jewels (Buddha, Dharma and Sangha), the Ten directions and of all times
>
> Myself and others, until we achieve enlightenment
>
> From my innermost heart, I take refuge in you

In the Buddhist tradition, there are different types of refuge:

- Sutra style, where you take refuge in Buddha, Dharma and Sangha
- Tantra style, where we take refuge in Guru, Deva and Dakini
- And another way is taking Inner refuge to our own potentiality, our own Buddhahood or Buddha-mind.

In the Yuthok Nyingthig we take refuge in Yuthok, in the union of Yuthok and Medicine Buddha.

We begin by visualising Yuthok as he appears on the Thangka before us. Although the outer form is Yuthok's, the quality is that of the Medicine Buddha which indicates that both are undividable, non-separated. Yuthok and Medicine Buddha are one. Then, we recite the refuge prayer in the Sutra style with awareness that the three objects of refuge, Buddha, Dharma and Sangha, are within Yuthok.

In the Tantra style, the Guru, Deva and Dakini are unified within Yuthok. In the Yuthok Nyingthig, as the quality of Yuthok's body and voice represent space in all existence, we can take refuge in nature and the five elements. So in the Yuthok Nyingthig style, we take refuge in natural medicine and our own self-potential or Buddhahood.

When we visualize Yuthok, we are actually imagining the Medicine Buddha whose colour is blue, representing infinite space with the quality of emptiness. When we take refuge in Yuthok or the Medicine Buddha, we should do so without boundaries; Yuthok represents the energy of the universe and we therefore take refuge in this natural universe. This is unique to the Yuthok Nyingthig style and it has to be understood that we must open our mind to the space without any boundaries.

If you take refuge in Buddhism that means that you choose to follow Buddha's steps. If you are a Buddhist you can take refuge in the Buddhist way, however as mentioned before, we can also take refuge in Yuthok and Medicine Buddha and their quality of natural medicine. Every flower can be a manifestation of Medicine Buddha and it exists for healing and balance.

In most Buddhist Mandalas, there are only Buddhist figures or deities however when we talk about the Medicine Buddha's Mandala, there are some non-Buddhist figures that are unique to this practice. For example, in the Mandala you find Shiva. So that when you take refuge in the Medicine Buddha, you also take refuge in Shiva. That doesn't mean that we take refuge in Buddhism and Hinduism. When we take refuge in the Medicine Buddha, we open our minds to the correct direction of healing, to help others with great love and ultimate compassion. Our taking refuge has no boundaries. It's important to help others and send out universal love and energy through Medicine Buddha and Yuthok's blessing.

We need to always be mindful that Medicine Buddha's Mandala is limitless and is therefore different to other Buddha's mandalas. Tibetan medicine is not only for Buddhists or for people of a particular nation, it is for everybody, every person and it is for this reason that Yuthok wished that Tibetan medicine would spread like the expanse of the sky, to help all beings. Thus, it's extremely important to take refuge in

Yuthok because through this, we can reach our ultimate goal as Yuthok promised us.

"If you give up your heart and mind to me
Beseech me in a sincere way
Overcome your lack of faith and
Hope in me as a refuge throughout your life
Immediately your two obscurations will diminish.
Upon meeting me in reality, in vision or in dream,
I will reveal the path to the temporal and ultimate goal."

Iconography of Yuthok

Typically in most traditions there is a refuge tree for the Ngöndro practice. However in the Yuthok Nyingthig practice, Yuthok represents all Buddha states and he does this in his common image.

In his right hand he holds an Uptala blossom, a blue Lotus flower, which represents Tara. Tara is known as the Action Buddha and so this symbolises that Yuthok is the union of all Buddha's actions (*rgyal kun 'phrin las gcig bsdus*).

Inside the flower, there is a text book or scroll and a sword which symbolise the Jamyang, meaning Yuthok has the wisdom of Jamyang, which is the Tibetan name for the Bodhisattva of Wisdom. Yuthok had a most extraordinary wisdom and memory, for example he memorised all Buddha's teachings and commentaries (*Bka' 'gyur bstan 'gyur*) as his song depicts.

"I explain the Buddhist canon and its commentaries by heart,
With logic I overcome the challenges of fundamentalists,
I issue the banner of victory of the Buddhist doctrine:
The title 'scholar' applies to me."

In his left hand, Yuthok holds a pink Lotus flower which represents *Chenrezig*, the Buddha of Compassion. This signifies that Yuthok has extraordinary compassion for all sentient beings. Inside the pink Lotus sits a Vase which is a representation of the Medicine Buddha and beside it is a Vajra which symbolises Vajrapani, telling us that Yuthok has Vajrapani's power and energy.

A Jewel sits on the Vase which is an image for wealth and represents Ratnasambava. Within this, there is also an Arura (or Myrobalan plant) which again signifies the Medicine Buddha. All together, these items represent the Five Buddha families. Known as the Five Dhyani Buddhas, they are icons of Mahayana Buddhism. Each represents a different aspect of enlightened consciousness to aid in spiritual transformation.

i.   **Akshobhya** is usually represented in blue. He is most often pictured touching the earth with his right hand, a gesture used by the historical Buddha when he asked the earth to bear witness to his enlightenment. In his left hand Akshobhya holds a vajra. The varja symbolises precision energy that is unstoppable, it transcends reality. In Buddhist tantra, evoking Akshobhya in meditation helps overcome anger and hatred.

ii. **Ratnasambhava Buddha** represents richness. His yellow or gold colour symbolizes the earth and he holds a wish-fulfilling jewel. He is sometimes referred to as the Buddha of Giving. Meditation on Ratnasambhava Buddha vanquishes pride.

iii. **Amitabha Buddha**'s name means infinite light, he is the colour of red, a colour associated with love and compassion and as such is known as the Buddha of Love and Compassion. Tantric meditation on Amitabha is an antidote to desire and greed. His symbol is the lotus, representing gentleness and purity.

iv. **Amoghasiddhi Buddha** holds a crossed vajra, a double dorje, representing accomplishment and fulfilment in all directions. He radiates a green light which indicates action and fearlessness. Meditation on Amoghasiddhi Buddha vanquishes envy.

v.   **Vairocana Buddha** whose name means illuminator is the bright white Buddha who resides in the centre of the mandala. His symbol is the Dharma wheel, which not only represents Buddhahood but Buddha's teachings which lead one to that Enlightenment state. His hand mudra represents the turning of the wheel. Meditation on Vairocana eliminates ignorance.

On Yuthok's head there sits a crown of five flowers symbolising five wisdoms or five Dakinis, and his white robe is a symbol of purity and the primordial state. Yuthok's long black hair, continually growing and never being cut off, is symbolic of his perfect knowledge and Dharma, and it also depicts him as a protector of medicine.

In this image, Yuthok's figure is the union of all Buddhas and we can see why Yuthok is called "All Buddhas in One Buddha" (*Gyel va kundus*). As Patrul Rinpoche mentions in his text 'Words of My Perfect Teacher':

> *"The teacher embodies the essence of all Buddhas throughout the three times, he is the union of the three jewels, his body is the sangha, his speech the Dharma, his mind the Buddha. He is the union of the three roots, his body is the teacher, his speech the yidam deity, his mind is the dakini, he is the union of the three kayas, his body is the nirmanakaya, his speech the sambhogakaya, his mind the dharmakaya.*
>
> *He is the embodiment of all the buddhas of the past, source of all the buddhas of future and the representative of all the buddhas of the present."*

It is important for us to focus on and understand that Yuthok holds the quality of Buddha, Dharma and Sangha, as well as Guru, Deva and Dakini.

One Tibetan master created a refuge tree for the Yuthok Nyingthig, for those who may find it easier for their visualisation. This can help as sometimes focusing on something visual can be more practical and easier and at the same time, help to remember the Guru's nature or quality. We should consider that Yuthok's body is a great treasure, one which is fulfilling all our desires.

Often people like to study different practices, each time they hear a new Buddha's name, they like to have it and feel they need that one too. But in the end they never achieve a single sound practice, since they are constantly changing their minds and desiring more. It is just like shopping, we would love to buy many things in a new market, and yet even after having bought many things we remain unsatisfied, still desiring more and more.

For this reason, it's very important to understand that doing the practice of one Buddha is better than doing ten different practices. When Atisha came to Tibet, he proclaimed "Tibetan people do practices of 100 Buddhas but haven't achieved one Buddha's blessing. It is much better to do the practice of one Buddha and once you have achieved that Buddha's siddhi, then you have achieved all Buddha's nature." This is a great and profound teaching.

So the idea of all Buddhas in one is very simple and in fact, it is the perfect Guru Yoga too. Keep the practice of your own one Buddha but respect all other Buddhas, then you can do their practices when there is a special need.

Yuthok's Prayer

The prayer beyond words (*Gangku Sang-chen-ma*)

This oldest and most known prayer to Yuthok was written by Sumtöng Yeshé Zung, Yuthok's heart disciple. When we read this prayer, it explains who Yuthok is, his supreme body, energy and mind. In this prayer, Sumtöng has captured the very essence of Yuthok. I love this prayer so much because this prayer is beyond words; in this prayer you can see and feel that Yuthok's energy is beyond all time and space, it has no boundary and his infinite blessing is always present with us.

The title *Gangku sang chen ma* means 'Whose Supreme Body or Whose Great Secret Body'. This prayer speaks about Yuthok's body, speech, mind knowledge and activities represented by his five chakras; the body chakra, throat, heart, navel and base chakra.

As mentioned earlier, this type of prayer or meditation is called Gyergom (*gyer bsgom*) which means chanting meditation. While we're chanting the prayer, we need to be aware of the meaning at the same time because concentrating the mind on the meaning is a kind of meditation in itself. Our mind is guided by chanting and this is an easy method to clear the mind and force it to concentrate. So we should not consider this prayer as a simple practice but as a specific kind of meditation.

The prayer consists of seven stanzas:

1) The Body of Yuthok, a non-destroyable nature

2) The Voice of Yuthok, roars of Dharma sounds

3) The Mind of Yuthok, a state of perfect wisdom

4) The Knowledge of Yuthok, the saviour of all beings

5) The Action of Yuthok, absolute liberation

6) The Calling of Yuthok, from the depth of the heart

7) The Summary of the prayer, the Supreme Mandala

Verse 1 – The Body of Yuthok, an indestructable nature

གང་གི་སྐུ་ཡི་གསང་ཆེན་མཆོག །

Gang gi ku yi sang chen chog
Whose supreme secret body,

དངོས་པོ་ཀུན་ཁྱབ་བདེ་བ་ཆེ། །

Ngö po kun kyab de wa che
Is the nature of Great Bliss that pervades all of existence,

རྣམ་ཀུན་མཆོག་ལྡན་རྡོ་རྗེའི་དབྱིངས། །

Nam kün chog den dorje ying
In all ways supremely endowed with the Vajra Realm.

མཚུངས་བྲལ་གུ་ཉའི་སྐུར་ཕྱག་འཚལ། །

Tsung dral gu nai kur chag tsel
To Yuthoks incomparable form, we prostrate

ན་མོ་གུ་རུ།

Na mo guru
Homage to the Guru

Whose supreme secret body
Is pervasive in all phenomenon with great bliss
At all times in supreme quality in the state of varja
(non-dualistic)
To Yuthoks incomparable body we prostrate

The first four lines of the prayer are in praise of Yuthok's body. They don't refer to his beauty or to our desire to have such a body, but to the mysterious quality of it, as can be discerned from the first line "*Whose supreme secret body*" (Gang gi ku yi sangchen chog).

The second line is also important as it talks about what Yuthok's body is and what is meant by the supreme body. *Ngö po kun kyab de va che* means that his body is omni-pervasive i.e. pervades or envelopes all phenomena.

When we talk about Yuthok's body, we're not referring to a painting or a *thangka* in front of us. We don't consider it in the form of a body like yours or mine. Instead, Yuthok's body exists in all phenomena, in each colour, in every manifestation. As mentioned before, Yuthok presented his teachings in his own distinctive way and that's why some aspects in the Yuthok Nyingthig differ from other teaching styles.

In Yuthok's song:

> *The illusory form of this body*
> *Is of the nature of a host of sacred deities;*
> *Its materiality is intrinsically pure.*
> *And like a rainbow, it cannot be grasped, yet*
> *Like the moon's reflection on the water, it appears everywhere.*

In Yuthok's teaching, a *guru* is not always a person; instead all existence can be a guru to us. A guru doesn't automatically imply that there will be teachings or mantra transmissions. A guru is not somebody who always guides or commands you. For us, our own life is the greatest guru. It is through life that we learn and understand so many things without words and explanations, where everything presented to us is in fact a teaching in itself.

For example a cup can be guru for us. When it breaks, we can understand the breaking of that cup and thereby recognize the nature of the cup. What that means is that its nature is impermanence and by it breaking, it has revealed its own nature. If we are able to understand the nature of impermanence by means of this cup then the cup has become our guru, it has perfectly displayed the nature of impermanence not by words, but by action.

In summary, Yuthok's body is not just a human body. The quality of Yuthok's body is found in all phenomena and existence, and like the energy of space, it is present in all existence.

The later part of the second line is *deva che* which means that in all existence, Yuthok's presence is inherent and it leads to joyfulness and bliss.

In the third line, the state of Vajra is non-duality, thus all existence is in the state of non-duality and is therefore un-destroyable.

Now on to the fourth line, *chag tsal* means that I do prostrations in front of Yuthok. Here, '*guna*' means the guru and '*tsung dral*' refers to his incomparable body.

These phrases actually represent some of the most important Buddhist philosophies that can be found in the Sutras; that form is emptiness and emptiness is form. Emptiness is the quality of the state of vajra which is the same quality as Yuthok's body and this explains why Yuthoks body is present in all phenomena.

Conclusively said Yuthoks body is emptiness, emptiness is form and form is emptiness. In the Tantras of the Vajrayana this is called *Nangtong* and means the non-separation between appearance and emptiness, which is the quality of Yuthok's body i.e. there is no difference between appearance and emptiness.

This is a form of prayer. Praying to Yuthok and being aware of the meaning is a direct link to emptiness. By understanding the qualities of Yuthok's body, we realize within our bodies the same qualities; that we ourselves are in the state of Vajra and emptiness.

Verse 2 - The Voice of Yuthok, roars of Dharma sounds

The next four sentences "*Sung*" is a prayer to Yuthok's voice.

གང་གི་གསུང་གི་གསང་ཆེན་མཆོག།

Gang gi sung gi sang chen chog
He whose supreme secret speech,

སྒྲ་གྲགས་ཀུན་ཁྱབ་གཞོམ་བྲལ་བ།།

Dra drak kün kyab shom drel wa
Is the indestructible quality that pervades all sound

བརྒྱད་ཁྲི་བཞི་སྟོང་ཆོས་སྒྲ་སྒྲོགས།།

Gye tri shi tong chö dra drog
Roaring the sound of the 84,000 dharmas,

མཚུངས་བྲལ་གུ་ནའི་གསུང་ཕྱག་འཚལ།།

Tsung dral gu nei sung chag tsal
To Yuthok's incomparable speech, we prostrate

Whose supreme secret speech
Is pervasive and indestructible in all sounds
He roars the 84,000 sounds of the dharma
To Yuthok's incomparable speech we prostrate

First there is the question of what is the supreme quality of Yuthok's speech. "*Sung*" is about Yuthok's voice energy being present in all kind of sounds. The Tibetan phrase *Dra drak kun kyab* means omni pervasive in all sounds and *Shomd del wa* means undestroyable. All these sounds resemble or teach the 84,000 voices or sounds of the dharma.

That means each sound we hear, each heartbeat, each breath, step etc represents a teaching of the dharma i.e. that everything is emptiness. All kinds of sounds are teaching us about impermanence and the nature of all existence is emptiness – that is the teaching of the 84,000 Dharmas. We have 84,000 emotions and Buddha's teaching is to balance all these emotions. But the basis of all these emotions is unawareness of the nature of the emptiness.

Thus any kind of sound, the sound of a river, a drop of water or music can be a guru to us and transmits something we can understand and realize.

In Yuthok's song:

> "*The empty sound of my voice is the song of the echo*
> *Reverberating with the sound of the 84,000 Dharmas,*
> *It manifests as a rain of teaching for those who need guidance,*
> *And sets all beings on the path that ripens and liberates.*"

In the Tantric teachings this is called *Dragtong Yerme (grags stong dbyer med)* which describes the non-separation between sound and emptiness. For example, one of the 84 enlightened *mahasiddhas* realized the quality of emptiness; his spiritual realization was achieved by listening to music that he loved. The sounds he listened to taught him about emptiness and in that way, music was his guru.

Another *mahasiddha* had a very precious stone in his ring which he was very fond of. He spent a lot of time looking at this special stone and somehow this stone made him understand what emptiness is and helped him to achieve spiritual enlightenment.

Verse 3 - The Mind of Yuthok, a state of perfect wisdom

The next four sentences are addressing his heart, or mind nature.

གང་གི་ཐུགས་ཀྱི་གསང་ཆེན་མཆོག །

Gang gi thüg kyi sang chen chog
He, whose supreme secret mind,

སྤྲོས་པ་ཀུན་བྲལ་བདེ་བ་ཆེ།།

Trö pa kün drel de wa che
Is unconditioned Great Bliss,

ཤེས་རབ་ཕ་རོལ་ཕྱིན་ལ་གནས།།

She rab pha rol chin la nei
Dwelling in the Perfection of Wisdom,

མཚུངས་བྲལ་གུ་ཊེའི་ཐུགས་ཕྱག་འཚལ།།

Tsung drel gu nai thüg chag tsal
To Yuthoks incomparable mind, we prostrate.

Whose supreme secret mind, (sky like in nature)
Exists without fabrications, always in bliss
In a state of perfect wisdom
To Yuthoks incomparable mind we prostrate.

The quality of Yuthok's heart is such that there are no fabrications, no limitations and no borders, it is like infinite space and the emptiness of that space is filled with great bliss.

The phrase *she rab pha rol chin la nei* describes the state of primordial wisdom, the highest state of consciousness. This state is like infinite space, which again is emptiness and bliss. To this, we offer prostrations to his heart.

In Yuthok's song:

> *"In the clarity and emptiness of my mind,*
> *the ineffable authentic state,*
>
> *Bliss is omni pervasive, arising unceasingly and,*
>
> *Emptiness and compassion are undifferentiated*
>
> *Hence, the phenomena created by mind are naturally liberated."*

Thus the nature of Yuthok's mind reminds us of our pure state of mind or awareness.

Verse 4 - The Knowledge of Yuthok, the saviour of all beings

The following four sentences deal with Yuthok's supreme knowledge.

རྒྱལ་བ་ཀུན་ཀྱང་འདྲེན་པ་ཁྱེད།།

Gyel wa kün kyang dren pa kye
You, who are the leader of all the Buddhas, entirely,

ཁྱེད་ལས་གཞན་པའི་སྐྱོབ་པ་ནི།།

Che le shen pai kyob pa ni
There is no refuge other than you

འགྲོ་བ་ཀུན་ལས་འགག་མ་མཆིས།།

Dro wa kün le gang ma chi
For all sentient beings;

དེ་ཕྱིར་ཁྱེད་ལ་སྐྱབས་སུ་མཆི།།

De chir che la kyab su chi
Because of this, in you I take refuge.

You, who are the leader of all the Buddhas
Beside you there is no other saviour
for all sentient beings
Peerless saviour
That is why I take refuge in you

This prayer to his knowledge is linked with the navel chakra, the chakra of manifestation. Through his supreme knowledge, Yuthok is leading and guiding all beings to a spiritual liberation that can only be achieved through the perfect union of wisdom and compassion. This knowledge refers to the supreme wisdom of understanding and experience of the state of emptiness in both subject and object.

The phrase *gyel wa kün kyang dren pa kye* means that Yuthok is the guidance of all Buddhas including the future Buddhas, and all those who will achieve liberation through Yuthok's practice and blessing. Yuthok safely leads all sentient beings, and that is why we take refuge in him. Yuthok has the knowledge and skill to liberate all sentient beings.

Verse 5 - The Action of Yuthok, absolute liberation

The next lines are concerned with Yuthok's actions.

ཕྱིས་པས་ཁྱེད་མཚན་མ་ཐོས་པ།།

Chi pe che tsen ma tö pam
Immature beings who haven't heard your name,

ཐོས་ཀྱང་གུས་པར་མི་བསྟེན་པ།།

Tö kyang gü par mi ten par
Or if they are able to hear your name but cannot be taught,

དེ་ལས་སྙིང་རྗེ་གཞན་མེད་པས།།

De le nying je shen me pe
For them, there is only compassion

བརྩེ་བའི་ཁྱེད་ཀྱིས་རྗེས་སུ་བཟུང་།།

Tse we kye kyi je su zung
Lead them with your loving kindness.

Beings or animals who don't know your name
Even when they hear your name they don't know how to follow you
We take compassion for all these sentient beings
Lead them with your compassion.

Yuthok's energy and blessing remains as long as space and beings remain, his particular action is helping beings to be liberated from pain and suffering.

Yuthok's presence is like a great sun with powerful energy. At times there may be places where sunlight is unable to reach, for instance in shadows. In those circumstances, it means there is no karmic connection to Yuthok. So, in this verse we're trying to make a connection with Yuthok and also to pray for those who have never seen or heard of Yuthok. Through this connection they can be blessed by Yuthok or Medicine Buddha and it is for this reason that we pray the following:

"We have compassion for all sentient beings who don't know how to follow him and pray that he helps them as well with his energies and blessings, which is Yuthok's action."

Yuthok's absolute liberation accomplishment is giving the path of rainbow body, which is the dissolvement of all the elements into pure emptiness.

Verse 6 – Calling Yuthok from the depth his heart

In the following we are taking refuge in Yuthok

ཁྱེད་ཀྱི་མཚན་ཐོས་སྐྱབས་སོང་བས།།

Che kyi tsän thö kyab song vei
Through hearing your name and taking refuge in you,

དེ་ནི་ནམ་ཡང་སྲིད་མཚོར་མིན།།

De ni nam yang si tsor min
They will no longer be in the ocean of Samsara.

དེ་ཕྱིར་མིག་ཆུ་ཡོ་བཞིན་དུ།།

De chir mik chu yo shin du
Because of this, with eyes filled with tears,

སྙིང་ནས་དུས་ཀུན་གསོལ་བ་འདེབས།།

Nying ni dü kün sol va deb
I pray to you at all times from my heart.

Hearing your name and taking refuge in you
Never again in the ocean of samsara
Therefore with eyes filled with tears
I always pray from my heart

Immediately after he finished writing the Four Medical Tantra, Yuthok received a vision of the Medicine Buddha and in that dream, three Buddha's prophesised that simply hearing the name of Yuthok, it would release a person from the depths of this samsaric ocean.

The three Buddhas said "Who see you, hear your name, think of you, touch you, have faith in you or even hate you, they will all achieve bliss, all beings will be blessed. You are the emanation of all, Yuthok. Who meditates on you, will be blessed. Yuthok will bless all who meditate on him."

When we pray to Yuthok, we need to know the meaning of the prayer and have faith in his supreme ability to lead and guide us. Our prayer should not only be performed verbally but from the very depths of our heart. This is of great importance.

It can be likened to getting water from a tap. If we want to get water, we have to open the tap otherwise the water will not flow. This is the same when we pray with our whole heart and faith. It is like opening the tap, where we can receive Yuthok's blessings. If we pray half-heartedly, it would be as though we're asking for the water to emit from the tap without opening it.

In many religions we often find reference to the term 'faith'. Some don't like this word, linking it to something very pious and holy with connotations of duty. Yet it is essential to generate complete trust and unfailing belief; faith can help us eliminate confusion and doubts and render the mind stable. When we don't believe in anything, there is no stable basis for the mind, no foundation for the mind to hold. No matter if it is a religious or spiritual belief, a faith of trust and positive awareness is a very important basis for many aspects of our lives; in times of difficulty or tragedy, our faith will keep our mind stable.

In some high levels of spiritual practice such as Vajrayana, one may falsely think that faith is not needed. In fact, no matter which practice we are involved in, faith is of most importance. It is through faith that we open ourselves up to blessings, energies and maybe even realisations.

In the Dzogchen tradition, known as the final great mind awareness (*rigpa*), it only can be achieved through perfect guru yoga; if there is no perfect faith there can be no perfect guru yoga.

And in the Mahamudra teachings, 100% pure faith is required in your Guru, his teachings and transmissions.

To explain further about faith, there is a story about the two Indian masters Naropa and Tilopa. Naropa followed Tilopa for twelve years, however Tilopa never taught him anything because he knew that Naropa was in fact a highly qualified Buddhist monk who had already studied all Buddhist philosophies. The reason why Tilopa made Naropa follow him for twelve years was to test his faith and devotion to his guru, to develop Naropa's faith to 100%. Even though Naropa was a most qualified Buddhist monk, he hadn't really experienced Mahamudra and the importance of faith. That's why Naropa gave up everything including his robes and monastery and followed Tilopa.

During that period, Naropa was asked by his master to do many stupid and dangerous things yet he performed them without even hesitating or contemplating if the tasks were life threatening or not. On a certain day, Tilopa saw Naropa's heart wide open, filled with 100% pure faith and devotion, when the transmission of Mahamudra is easier.

So, Tilopa took off his shoes and slapped Naropa on his head... and that was it! Tilopa said to him:

> "The self nature wisdom is beyond of words and voice
> I (Tilopa) have nothing to show you,
> The nature of your own mind - naked wisdom
> you should know by yourself."

Those were his words of transmission which led to Naropa's enlightenment. Conclusively, having faith is like opening the heart completely and by means of this devotion, blessings can enter into us.

Yuthok says that if there is the right moment for the perfect master and the karmic disciple, one is open completely and the other gives completely, then realization happens in that one instance or moment.

Verse 7 – Prayer summary, the Supreme Mandala

རབ་འབྱམས་རྒྱལ་བའི་དཀྱིལ་འཁོར་མཆོག །

Rab jam gyal wai kyil kor chog
Infinite supreme mandalas of the Buddhas,

གསང་ཆེན་ཁྱེད་སྐུར་རོ་གཅིག་པ །

Sang chen che kur ro chig pe
Are 'one taste' to your supreme body

དེ་རིང་ཁོ་ནར་མངོན་སུམ་དུ །

De ring kho nar ngön sum du
Today, right now and in actuality,

མཁའ་ཁྱབ་འགྲོ་བའ་ཐོབ་པར་ཤོག །

Kha chab dro we tob par shog
May all sentient beings pervading space attain this.

Countless Buddha's supreme Mandala
Exactly the same as your supreme body
Today, here in reality
All sentient beings may achieve it

In the last four lines of the prayer the countless mandalas of the Buddhas are mentioned. It mentions that they are of the "same taste" as Yuthok's body which simply means that they are exactly the same.

We have the Medicine Buddha, Compassion Buddha, Wisdom Buddha, Wealth Buddha, and Activity Buddha and so on; countless Buddhas which all have qualities that are unified and which can be found in the one who is Yuthok.

De ring kho nar is the pledge that Yuthok shall use his energies and power here, today and right now. Further on, we pray that all sentient beings shall receive Yuthok's power and blessings. We no longer pray to Yuthok just on behalf of ourselves or the resolution of our personal problems but for all sentient beings that they may attain his blessing.

As a summary:

Yuthok's body is the union of appearance and emptiness

Yuthok's speech is union of sound and emptiness

Yuthok's mind is union of great bliss and emptiness

His knowledge leads all Buddhas and his action is liberating all beings

from Samsara He is a manifestation of all Buddha's action.

Bodhicitta and the Four Immeasurables

The Mahayana Bodhicitta practice of compassion, aspiration and entering.

སངས་རྒྱས་ཆོས་དང་ཚོགས་ཀྱི་མཆོག་རྣམས་ལ།

Sang-ye chö dang tshog kyi chog nam la
The Buddha, dharma and supreme assembly (sangha),

བྱང་ཆུབ་བར་དུ་བདག་ནི་སྐྱབས་སུ་མཆི།།

Chang chub bar du dag ni kyab su chi
Until enlightenment I take refuge in you,

བདག་གིས་སྦྱིན་སོགས་བགྱིས་པའི་བསོད་ནམས་ཀྱིས།།

Dag gi jin-sog gyi-pai sö nam kyi

I will, through the merit of generosity and so on,

འགྲོ་ལ་ཕན་ཕྱིར་སངས་རྒྱས་འགྲུབ་པར་ཤོག།།

Dro-la pen chir sang gye drub par shog

Achieve Buddhahood for the benefit of all sentient beings.

In the first sentence, *sang-ye* means Buddha and here it refers to Medicine Buddha. The word *cho* means Dharma and in this context it refers to the Medicine Buddha and Yuthok's teachings.

The phrase *tsog kyi chog* refers to Bodhisattvas such as Chenrezig, Jamyang, Tara etc. and it is also refers to Medicine Dakinis and Rishis.

Chin sog refers to the six perfections:

1. Generosity – perfect generosity, able to give all

2. Ethics or morality – perfect morality

3. Patience – perfection of patience for practicing

4. Effort – perfection of effort for helping others

5. Meditations – perfection of meditation

6. Wisdom – perfection of wisdom is realization of self nature

Bodhichitta has two main meanings; one is compassion and other is the enlightened mind, or a purified perfected mind. In fact, these two meanings are interdependent because in order to achieve an enlightened mind we must have the basis of compassion.

There are two aspects to Bodhichitta; Relative Bodhichitta and Absolute Bodhichitta.

Relative Bodhichitta means that we use compassion and love for helping others and has two stages; the first stage is called *monsem* (*sMon Sems*), thinking positively or to have a good intention and the second is acting or working with compassion. It's not enough that we just have good intention; we must act on it and practice it too. So the first stage is about understanding and mental preparation and the second one is about integrity with the actual practice.

Absolute Bodhichitta is the self-realization of our own mind, in other words obtaining the perfect mind.

The text that we use in the Yuthok Nyingthig practice to generate Bodhichitta is a standard one taken from Buddhist sutras. Again we find Buddha, Dharma and Sangha, which is typical sutra style but as mentioned, they all are present in Yuthok.

Apart from two aspects, there are also two types of Bodhichitta. The first is that we wish and desire to help others however it may not be possible to do it physically so we do it mentally. That means, even if we're not able to treat or to help someone physically, we can still wish the best for a person and generate a positive motivation.

For the second type, we are not only thinking and wishing but also taking action. According to Yuthok, performing any healing work or indeed any activity to help others with compassion is practising the action of Bodhichitta. Yuthok said that he chose medicine because he knew how to use his hands to remove people's suffering and pain directly and thus went to the practical part of Bodhichitta. That is the main reason why he did not focus so much on the other Buddha Dharma practice.

The Four Immeasurables – the universal compassion

An immeasurable heart and mind with infinite love.

Sem-chen tam-chay de-wa-dang
de-way gyu-dang den-par-gyur-chig

Sem-chen tam-chay dug-ngel-dang
dug-ngel-kyi gyen-dang delwar gyur-chig

Sem-chen tam-chay dug-ngel me-pay
dewa-dang mi-drel-war gyur-chig

Sem-chen tam-chay nye-ring chag-dang nyi-dang
drel-way-thang nyom-la nay-par gyur-chig

Translation of the Four Immeasurables prayer:

i.   **Immeasurable Love** - May all beings have happiness and the causes of happiness

ii. **Immeasurable Compassion** - May all beings be free from suffering and the causes of suffering

iii. **Immeasurable Joy** - May all beings never be separated from the supreme joy that is beyond all sorrow

iv. **Immeasurable Equanimity** - May all beings abide in a state of equanimity, free from attachment, aversion and sorrow

This prayer is quite a common prayer and can easily be found in the sutra texts and other texts as well. Because of its commonality, many people think it's a just simple prayer and often don't consider the meaning behind it. In fact, this prayer is at the heart of spiritual practice. It is simple but profound, easy yet complex, short yet beautiful. In its simplicity, it conveys absolute spirituality.

The first line stands for immeasurable love, a perfect love for all sentient beings. The second is about immeasurable compassion, a universal compassion for all sentient beings. The third prays for immeasurable joy and infinite happiness for all sentient beings. The fourth and final line is about immeasurable equanimity, absolute serenity for all sentient beings.

Why are they called immeasurable? Why can't these aspirations be measured? If our love is limited i.e. we only love one person or a few people, then it is measured, limited. But if we love countless beings irrespective of who they are, then our mind and love are infinite, it cannot be measured. The true quality of love and compassion cannot be limited.

If we consider the quality of our mind as a space without a centre and with directions beyond limitations and conditions, and if we send love with this quality of our mind, the quality of the love we send will have the same quality as our mind i.e. limitless. Take an electric light for example. In most houses light is available, you just have to switch the button to turn it on, but we're not aware of how the electricity is harnessed to generate the light in the home. Similarly, the physical heart is a piece of muscle full of blood vessels, it beats and gives us life, it can be transplanted by surgery, it can be measured and weighed, however it's extraordinary hidden nature is absolutely beyond any limitations.

Every mind is full of infinite, countless love and compassion – push the button to activate it and let it flow. Don't close your heart, don't set self-limitations, just open your immeasurable heart and feel it's potentiality, think of all and love all from the depth of your heart.

Since the mind creates everything, we can generate good motivation by employing positive thoughts. This mind quality can be present in all phenomena and all sentient beings. Yuthok repeats one sentence in his teachings saying "all phenomena should stay at one point or tip of your mind". Every manifestation is a creation of our mind. Every single thought is an energy or vibration, it creates or effects different parts of phenomena; when we generate positive thought, it can benefit beings who are in need. That energy remains in the universe and will continue to spontaneously affect others, even after our death.

The potential of our mind is to send love to all sentient beings, giving them love, kindness and happiness; we should not just limit this to individual patients we encounter through our medical practice.

Some spiritual practitioners might laugh when being confronted by these terms of love, compassion, happiness and equanimity. They feel these words are too simple and not the way to spiritual enlightenment. Some practitioners may say that they do for example, a special mantra or visualization of a deity, chant or sing something, take a particular meditation position, have visions and magic powers which may be considered as the highest and most special spiritual practices. But I ask, what is the aim of a Buddhist spiritual practice? The main question here is, are you doing the practice for yourself or for others? If it is only for you, then there is no base of Bodhicitta and compassion because by thinking only of ourselves, we are not opening our heart and mind; without opening the mind, we can never reach spiritual realisation.

If someone does a spiritual practice to calm their own mind or for comfort and that is his or her main aim, then it's fine. This person is just looking for a simple free mind for self, but it is a self-limited practice. The root of Buddhist tradition is to include all sentient beings and give them our love, compassion, happiness and equanimity. Without this root even a very powerful mantra or an elaborate meditation technique remains self-impressing and lacks the right aim.

There is a Tibetan word 'Randrol' (rang grol) which means self liberation, except this is not liberation only for the self. Self liberation here means helping others, self liberation is realization of ones self mind nature which, once obtained, is used to help others reach realisation too. But without basic virtue or compassion, no practice can help you reach it. If you bring your spiritual practice into real life and try to integrate it with an understanding of why you are practising, then you will need the Four Immeasurables as your foundation. Without this direction and intention, there is no sense in the practice.

In my experience, I believe that positive thought is the beginning of positive action, and that is the main cause of positive result.

Most people like the idea of doing a secret or higher spiritual practice, yet they should not lose the most important motivation for following their chosen practice. If someone becomes a Buddha, then what do they do? If someone achieves a rainbow body, what's next? After becoming a Buddha, he or she should work like other Buddhas, and do you know what the main is practice is then? The Four Immeasurables!

How to do this practice

Sit comfortably, breathe slowly and deeply. Read the text and think of its meaning, but really feel it. Make sure your intention of the meaning is clear and strong.

The practice is best in the early morning or evening, or any time in your life. It should take from 5 to 10 minutes. Don't leave it to just reading the prayer, don't just rest in the words. Try to do some virtuous actions as well without thinking too much about it.

Prostrations – Purification of the Body

This is a movement meditation which purifies our body. When the body is purified, blessings flow in the channels perfectly. It is a purification of the body through a simple yoga.

These four lines are a prayer to our guru Yuthok.

"From whose kindness, the great bliss (liberation)
Instantly arises inside of us
Lama, the precious guru,
The vajra holder, I prostrate to you."

Yuthok said "If a qualified master meets a karmic disciple, then the spiritual realisation can be achieved in an instant". This is the reason why we do prostrations to Yuthok, so that through his blessing we can achieve liberation.

The Tibetan word *chagtsel* means prostrations. Prostrations are a very simple type of Tibetan yoga and may be compared to the Indian yoga tradition called 'Salute to the Sun'. In Tibetan, *'chag'* means hand and *'tsel'* means moving, so it can be translated as 'hand movement yoga'. Many Tibetans love to do this practice and it's the most typical form of physical exercise.

If we look closely, prostrations have four fundamental benefits:

- Physical benefit
- Energetic benefit
- Mental benefit
- Spiritual benefit

On a physiological aspect, prostrations are an important and beneficial physical exercise which helps our digestive system, helps to increase our metabolism and energies, supports good blood circulation and loss of weight. Prostrations can also help to shift negative thoughts.

On the energetic level, prostrations are a basic movement that can unblock many knots in our channels. According to the Vajrayana tradition, the more knots we have in our anatomy the more emotional disturbances and sicknesses we suffer. That's why many yogic exercises are especially aimed at unblocking these energetic blockages.

Mentally, negative emotions can be expelled during the prostration, and clarity of mind is the result.

On the spiritual level there are three different beneficial aspects. The first is to pacify and diminish our ego and pride by bowing down in front of Yuthok. Secondly, the movement of going up and down is a metaphor for the ups and downs of our lives and represents our ability to escape a life in samsara. Thirdly while prostrating, we visualize all sentient beings doing the same and thereby establish a karmic connection between them, Yuthok and the Medicine Buddha.

To feel comfortable when doing this practice, it's important to be aware of the healthy, energetic, emotion and spiritual benefits and value of the prostrations. Otherwise, it just becomes a physical exercise without any deeper understanding.

Mandala Offering and Circumambulation

Mandala Offering – Perfect Generosity

This is a meditation founded on generosity; physically we offer the symbolic mandala but mentally we offer the whole universe.

In the tradition, there are three types of mandala offerings:

1. The ordinary mandala of the **Nirmanakaya**. This is offering all things to which we are mentally attached in our life like our loved ones, fortune, wealth, power, strength, life itself and so on.

2. The extraordinary mandala of the **Sambhogakaya**. This is offering the five perfections:
    *   Perfect location - pure dimension
    *   Perfect guru - five Buddha families
    *   Perfect assembly - bodhisattvas
    *   Perfect teaching - pure teachings of medicine and great Buddha dharma
    *   Perfect time - an ever-revolving wheel of eternity

    It also includes our pure vajra body, pure energy and primal wisdom.

3. The special all pervading mandala of the **Dharmakaya**. This refers to the offering of the pure aspect of the mind. All phenomena are a display of our primordial wisdom, a spontaneous presence which is beyond pure and impure or existence or non-existence. A perfect and spontaneous mind is the greatest offering to the

absolute guru Yuthok.

In order to realise inner knowledge and to accumulate the two merits (giving and receiving), this is the common mandala for training our mind. The prayer associated with the offering is given below.

བདག་གཞན་ལུས་དང་ལོངས་སྤྱོད་དུས་གསུམ་གྱི།།

Dag shen lü dang long chö dü sum gyi
The body, possessions and pleasures of myself and others,
of the three times,

དགེ་ཚོགས་དང་བཅས་རི་རྒྱལ་ཉི་ཟླ་སོགས།།

Ge tsog dang che ri ling nyi da sog
And all accumulations virtues, together with Mount Meru,
the Four continents, the sun and moon and so on.

ཀུན་བཟང་མཆོད་སྤྲིན་བསམ་ཡས་སྤྲུལ་བྱས་ཏེ།།

Kun zang chö trin sam ye trül jehteh
The emanated inconceivable offering clouds of Kuntuzangpo,

བླ་མ་དཀོན་མཆོག་ཐུགས་རྗེ་ཅན་ལ་འབུལ།།

La ma kön chog thük je chen la bül
I offer to the compassionate Lama, the Three Jewels

བསོད་ནམས་ཡེ་ཤེས་ཚོགས་གཉིས་རྫོགས་པར་ཤོག།

Sö nam ye shay tsok nyi dzog par shog
May the two accumulations of merit and wisdom be perfected.

My body and all belongings and others too, of the three times,
All virtues, Mount Meru, the four lands, the sun and moon,
The ultimate and infinite perfect offerings,
I offer to the precious Guru who is filled with compassion,
May the two merits (common & wisdom merit) be achieved

As explained in the last sentence of the prayer, the reason for offering the mandala is to accumulate the relative common merit and the absolute merit or wisdom. In this practice, the abundance of the offering is of significant importance. As described in the first lines, we offer not only our bodies but also that of other beings and all belongings of the three times, the past, present and future. We offer all accumulated good virtues and merit, we offer Mount Meru, all the Continents and the Sun and Moon. In other words, we're offering the whole universe to Yuthok or the Medicine Buddha. This is regarded as an exercise to open the mind and not withhold anything for ourselves but to give everything to Yuthok.

The principal idea is that the more we offer to the universe the more we get back. If you want to receive positive energy, wisdom and prosperity, you first have to offer everything. Then the universe responds by giving us what we need in a spontaneous way. In this context, the universe is actually Yuthok's presence or energy, so the mandala offering is all about giving and receiving - the more you give the more you receive.

There are also many rituals and practices concerning material aspects like increasing wealth by employing the power of special deities. Yet when you delve into the meaning of all these different practices, you'll find the base always relates to the offering of a mandala. No mantra or other spiritual practice could help to accumulate the infinite merit more spontaneously than offering a mandala.

Imagine yourself as a drop of water and offering yourself to the ocean. Your existence would continue for as long as that of the ocean. However if we become separated from the ocean, we remain just a drop of water which can be easily dried up. In this practice, by offering ourselves and everything without boundaries to the universe, we become part of and merge into it. This offering attracts prosperity which will reach the universe and as we are the universe, we will benefit as well.

When doing the offering we can use the rice mandala with the metal bowl or apply the *mudra* of Mount Meru. Turning around clockwise three times symbolizes offering, anticlockwise is for receiving. Then, release the *mudra* and start over again. At a certain location on the wrist, we have a special channel which opens with the help of this technique, unblocking our attachments and allowing us to receive universal energy and blessing.

Circumambulation – Purification of Channels

This is a walking meditation, keeping our mind focus on the steps as we walk.

Korwa (*bsKor ba*) means circumambulation; it is an important physical exercise. It mainly refers to walking meditation or walking with mindfulness. Every year, we take millions of steps and sometimes it's good to take these steps with mindfulness or intention and take peaceful steps for others. It is for this reason that Yuthok mentioned that circumambulation should be done with Ngöndro.

In our practice, we now see two physical aspects, prostrations and circumambulation; but the latter are only practiced in the Yuthok Nyingthig, and not included in other types of Ngöndro. As with prostrations, circumambulation is a practice that improves physical health, releases emotions and calms the mind, unblocking energy channels and spiritually brings a blessing from Yuthok or Medicine Buddha.

While performing circumambulation, visualize all sentient beings doing the same, thereby establishing a karmic connection between them, Yuthok and the Medicine Buddha.

We recite the short version of the Medicine Buddha Mantra:

Tayata Om
Bhe-kha-dze Bhe-kha-dze
Ma-ha Bhe-kha-dze
Raza Samud-Gate So-ha.

In Sanskrit:

Tadyatha Om
Bheshajae Bheshajae
Ma ha Bhe sha zae
Raja Samud Gate Svaha.

Translation:

Medicine Buddha, Medicine Buddha,
Great Medicine Buddha,
King of the Awakened,
Bless me.

We recite this mantra while performing one hundred and one circumambulations around the mandala, visualizing all sentient beings with us, and Medicine Buddha granting his ultimate blessing.

The Benefits of Medicine Buddha Practice

According to the Medicine Buddha Sutra, upon attaining Enlightenment, the Medicine Buddha announced Twelve Vows:

1. To illuminate countless realms with his radiance, enabling anyone to become a Buddha.

2. To awaken the minds of sentient beings through his energy.

3. To provide sentient beings with whatever material needs they

require.

4. To correct heretical views and inspire beings toward the path of the Buddha

5. To help beings follow the Moral and positive Precepts.

6. To heal beings born with deformities, illness or other physical sufferings.

7. To help relieve the destitute and the sick.

8. To help sentient beings achieve a desired rebirth.

9. To help heal mental afflictions and delusions.

10. To help free the oppressed from suffering.

11. To relieve those who suffer from terrible hunger and thirst.

12. To help clothe those who are destitute and suffering from the cold.

In Vajrayana or Tantra traditions, the Medicine Buddha practice is not only a powerful method for healing both oneself and others, but also for overcoming the inner afflictions of attachment, hatred, ignorance, ego and jealousy. The Medicine Buddha mantra can help decrease physical and mental illness and suffering, as well as the purification of negative or bad karma. By practicing the Medicine Buddha meditation, one has the opportunity to eventually attain spiritual enlightenment as well.

Purification – Vajrasattva Practice (*Dor-sem*)

རྡོར་སེམས་བསྐོམ་སྒྲུབ།

In Tibetan, *Dorje* means Vajra which represents a non-duality or un-destroyable nature. *Sempa* means the warrior of mind. *Dorje Sempa* or Dor-Sem simply means Vajrasattva is the un-destroyable mind warrior. The Buddha who is the un-destroyable mental warrior can purify all our negativities so we follow this practice to purify our selves.

Vajrasattva's prayer:

རང་གི་སྤྱི་བོར་པད་ཟླའི་སྟེང་།།
Rang gi chi wor pe dai teng
Above my head in a white lotus moon disc

ཧཱུྃ་དཀར་ལས་གྲུབ་རྡོ་རྗེ་སེམས།།
Hung kar lei drub Dorje Sem
On which a white Hung becomes Vajrasattva

ལོངས་སྤྱོད་རྫོགས་སྐུའི་ཆ་ལུགས་ཅན།།
Long chö dzok kui cha lug chen
In manner and accoutrements of Samboghakaya,

ཕྱག་གཉིས་རྡོ་རྗེ་དྲིལ་བུ་འཛིན།།
Chak nyi dorje drilbu dzin
The two hands holding vajra and bell.

ཐུགས་ཀར་ཟླ་སྟེང་ཧཱུྃ་གི་མཐར།།
Thük kar da ting Hung gi thar
At his heart is a moon disc with the syllable Hung,

ཡི་གེ་བརྒྱ་བའི་སྔགས་ཀྱིས་བསྐོར།།
Yi ge gya pai ngag kyi kor
Surrounded by the hundred syllable mantra

འོད་འཕྲོས་འཕགས་མཆོད་འགྲོ་དོན་བྱས།།
Ö trö phag chö dro dön jeh
Which radiates light which offers to the Buddhas and benefits sentient beings.

བདུད་རྩི་མཐེབ་སོར་ནས་འཛག་པས།།

Dütsi theb sor ne dzag pai
Nectar pours from Vajrasattva's big toe,

རང་གི་ལུས་བགྲུས་སྡིག་སྒྲིབ་ཀུན།།

Rang gi lü tru dig drib kün
Washing through my body; All stains and obscurations

མ་ལུས་བྱང་ཞིང་དག་པར་གྱུར།།

Ma lü chang shing dag par gyur
With exception are completely cleansed and become purified.

The translation is:

> Above my head in a white lotus moon disc
> White 'Hung' is transformed to Vajrasattva
> He is in the form of Samboghakaya
> Two hands holding vajra and bell
> At his heart there is a moon disc with the letter 'Hung'
> The letter is surrounded by the hundred syllable mantra
> Radiating light offers to the Buddhas and purifies sentient beings
> Nectar pours from Vajrasattva's big toe
> Washing my body and all negativities
> Completely cleaned and purified.

To be a good doctor, healer or practitioner, it is imperative to cleanse our body's channels and our mind's poisons. We need to purify negative energy and bad karma and the most effective and efficient way to do that is the practice of Dorje Sempa. Yuthok taught that, at any time when you have a free moment, it is a good opportunity to do the Dor-sem practice, to purify all negativities.

There are four stages to the Vajrasattva practice:

- Visualise the Dor-sem Buddha
- Think of any bad actions we have done with regret
- Promise to never do it again
- Purify bad karma and energies or action

When we recite the prayer, we visualise nectar as a liquid or light entering and purifying our bodies, our bad karma, sicknesses, diseases and bad energies. The most important point here is that Dor-sem is non-separated from Yuthok, Dor-sem is Yuthok. The short mantra is:

Sanskrit: Om Vajrasattva Hum
Tibetan: Om Bezar Sato Hung

It simply translates as "Vajrasattva, the mind warrior Buddha, bless me". The long mantra is known as the '100 Syllable Purification Mantra':

Om Vajrasattva Samaya Ma Nu Palaya
Vajrasattva Tenopa Tishda Dri-dho Me Bhava
Suto-shayo Me Bhava Supo-shayo Me Bhava
Anu-rakto Me Bhava Sarva siddhi Me Pra-ya-tsa
Sarva Karma Sutsa Me Tsitam Shre-yam Kuru-hum
Ha Ha Ha Ha Ho!
Bhagavan Sarva Tathagata Vajra Ma-me Muntsa
Vajra Bhava Maha Samaya Sattva
Ah Hung Phat

The meaning of the long mantra is:

Om Vajrasattva, preserve the bond!
As Vajrasattva, stand before me
Be firm for me
Be greatly pleased for me
Deeply nourish me
Love me passionately
Grant me siddhi in all things
And in all actions make my mind most excellent. Hum!
Ha Ha Ha Ha Ho!
Blessed one, Vajra of all the Tathagatas,
do not abandon me
Be the Vajra-bearer, the being of the Great Bond!
Ah Hung Phat

Key Points of the practice
There are three main stages of purification.

1. To purify the physical body, visualise the following:

    The nectar pours from Dor-sem's toes in a stream and enters our skull via our crown, then travels into the brain, the sense organs, to the neck, the trunk, all organs, the lungs, heart, liver, spleen, pancreas, kidneys, the stomach, gallbladder, small intestine, colon, then shoulders, arms, hand and fingers. Then to the hips, thighs, legs, feet and toes. From skin to muscles, blood vessels, blood, tendons, bones, bone marrow; then it cleans every cell and micro-organism, cleans all bad energy or sickness and comes out from the nine orifices; the eyes, ears, nose, mouth, anus, urine orifice and as well as from every single pore.

This bad energy comes out in the form of black fluid, smoke or dirty water. Once this bad energy exits, it transmutes into a positive energy for nature, then dissolves into nature or space.

2. To purify the energy, visualise:

The nectar enters from the central Channel and travels to the right and left Channels, then it enters the chakras. From there, the nectar enters the entire body's countless Channels and having purified them completely, the band of energy leaves the body in the form of black smoke or brown air.

3. To purify mental emotion, you should visualise:

The nectar enters as a light and when it touches our head, our whole body is lit with an extraordinary energy light. At this point, all our emotions are like the darkness and the wisdom light expels them immediately. The mind's state remains very clear and all ignorance is purified; then our anger, attachment, pride and jealousy are dissolved in the light too. If you have any particular emotion, the light of this nectar can eliminate it.

Finally, our body, energy and mind are perfectly purified and we see ourselves as a pure and bright crystal. Then Vajrasattva dissolves into us and we are self transformed into Vajrasattva, the surrounding dimension becomes his mandala, mindfulness on the pure dimension.

At the end all dissolves into the space or emptiness and we rest in the state of absolute emptiness.

Kusali – the Perfect Body Offering

This practice of offering the body is based on the Tibetan practice of *chöd*. This was generated by the famous Tibetan female practitioner Machik Labdron (1031—1129).

The meaning of *chöd* is cutting and refers to the cutting away of fear and attachment. The Tibetan *chöd* practice is a complete and elaborate system in itself. In contrast, the *Kusali* practice is a more simplified way of achieving the body offering practice. The aim of this practice is to transform our bodies into nectar or light and to offer this nectar or light body to all sentient beings.

A typical aspect of *chöd* is the elimination of the four types of demons. Of course this is not physically fighting actual demons. It refers to the mental and psychological obstacles in our lives and on the path of spiritual enlightenment.

According to the treatise "Words of my Perfect Teacher" by the great Patrul Rinpoche, we can dispel the Four Demons, inside and outside:

"What we call demon is not something with gaping jaws and glaring eyes; rather it is that which creates all the afflictions of Samsara and prevents the attainment of liberation, the state of nirvana. In short it is anything that harms (or afflicts) one's body and mind."

The Four Demons are:

1. *The Demon of the Aggregates*; is the base of suffering and creates many obstacles on our spiritual path.

2. *The Demon of Negative* emotions; is the base of all Samsara. When we lose control of our emotions they bring out the worst in us like anger, hate, pride, jealousy and so on, all of these can bring samsaric pain and suffering. In this way, even our limited love and good emotions can become the cause of bad effects.

3. *The Demon of the Death*; early death is an obstacle of the spiritual path as we need a certain amount of time before we can achieve enlightenment.

4. *The Demon of Illusion*; leads us towards the wrong path. In our normal life there are so many distractions and all are simply manifestations of our illusions. If we believe in them, they can be obstacles for our spiritual journey.

Chöd relates to cutting three types of obstacles:

- External Obstacles - fear and emotions are related to environment
- Internal Obstacles - is attachment to self and body
- Secret Obstacles - are ignorance of mind or unawareness of the true nature of self

Kusali Body Offering Practice

ཀུ་ས་ལི། ལུས་སྦྱིན།

མདུན་མཁར་བླ་མ་སྨན་པའི་རྒྱལ་པོ་ལ།།
Dün kar lama man pai gyal po la
In the sky in front is the lama, King of Medicine,

མགྲོན་རིགས་བཞིས་བསྐོར་སྤྲིན་ཕུང་གཏིབ་ལྟར་བཞུགས།།

Drön rig shi kor trin pung tib tar shuk
Residing amidst the four classes of guests, like a massed gathering of clouds,

རང་སེམས་དབྱིངས་སྟོན་རྡོ་རྗེ་རྣལ་འབྱོར་མ།།

Rang sem ying tön Dorje Naljorma
One's own consciousness is ejected into space,

དམར་མོ་གྲི་ཐོད་འཛིན་པའི་སྐུ་རུ་གྱུར།།

Mar mo dri tö dzin pai ku ru gyur
Becoming the form of Vajrayogini,
holding a curved knife and skull cap,

བེམ་པོའི་ཐོད་པ་ཕྱག་གཡས་གྲི་གུག་གིས།།

Bem poi thö pa chak ye dri gug gi
With her driguk, she cuts open the skull of our corpse,

བྲེགས་ཏེ་རང་བྱུང་ཐོད་པའི་སྒྱེད་པུར་བཙུགས།།

Dreg te rang chung thö pai gyed pur tsug
Placing it on a self-arisen hearth of skulls,

དེ་ནང་ཤ་རུས་ཏིལ་འབྲུ་ཚམ་དུ་བསིལ།།

De nang sha rü til dru tsam du sil
Inside the skull, the flesh and bones are chopped fine as mustard seeds,

མེ་རླུང་སྦྱོར་བའི་ཟགས་མེད་བདུད་རྩིའི་མཚོ།།

Me lung jor vei sag med düd tsi tso
Through conjoined fire and wind, it becomes an inexhaustible ocean of nectar,

ནམ་མཁའི་ཁྱོན་གང་མཆོད་སྤྲིན་ཟད་མི་ཤེས།།

Nam khai kyön gang chö trin ze mi shay
Filling the breadth of space with endless offering clouds,

མགྲོན་རིགས་སོ་སོའི་འདོད་ཞེས་རྒུར་འཆར་བར་གྱུར།།

Drön rig so soi shay gur char var gyur
Whatever is wished for or desired arises for each class of guest,

ཐུགས་ལས་མཆོད་པའི་ལྷ་མོ་གྲངས་མེད་སྤྲོས།།

Thuk leh chö pai lhamo drang meh trö
Through countless offering goddesses emanated from the heart of Vajrayogini,

ༀ་ཨཱ་ཧཱུྃ།

Om Ah Hung (Repeat 101 times)

དཀོན་མཆོག་རྩ་གསུམ་སྲིད་ཞིའི་མགྲོན་རྣམས་ལ།།

Kön chog tsa sum si shui drön nam la
The Three Jewels and Three Roots, guests of apparent existence,

གུས་པས་འབུལ་ལོ་ཚོགས་གཉིས་ཛོ་གས་པར་ཤོག།

Gü pei bul lo tsog nyi nyur dzog shog
Offering with devotion to perfect the two accumulations,

དཔལ་མགོན་ཆོས་སྐྱོང་ཡོན་ཏན་མགྲོན་རྣམས་ལ།།

Pal gön chö kyong yön ten drön nam la
Glorious dharma protectors, the Guests of Quality,

འབུལ་ལོ་ལས་དང་དངོས་གྲུབ་འགྲུབ་པར་མཛོད།།

Bül lo le dang ngö drub drub par dzö
Through offering to you, perform activity and grant siddhi,

འགྲོ་བ་རིགས་དྲུག་སྙིང་རྗེའི་མགྲོན་རྣམས་ལ།།

Dro wa rig druk nying jei drön nam la
Beings of the six realms, Guests of Compassion,

སྦྱིན་པས་སྡུག་བསྔལ་ཀུན་ཞི་བདེ་ལྡན་ཤོག།
Jin pe dug ngel kün shi de den shog
Through generosity, may your suffering be pacified and may you have happiness,

སྡེ་བརྒྱད་འབྱུང་པོ་ལན་ཆགས་མགྲོན་རྣམས་ལ།།
De gye jung po len chak drön nam la
The eight classes of Elementals, the Karmic Debtor Guests,

བསྔོས་པས་ཞི་བ་བྱང་ཆུབ་སེམས་ལྡན་ཤོག།
Ngö pe shi wa chang chub sem den shog
By dedicating to you, may you possess the mind of Bodhicitta,

ཀུན་ཀྱང་རིག་འདུས་བླ་མའི་ཡེ་ཤེས་ཀྱི།།
Kün kyang rig dü lamai ye shay kyi
Through the wisdom of the lamas and knowledge-holders,

སྒྱུ་འཕྲུལ་རོལ་པ་ཅིར་ཡང་སྣང་བ་སྟེ།།
Gyu trul rol pa chir yang nang wa teh
And the illusory play of appearances,

ལུས་ཀྱི་མཆོད་སྦྱིན་ཕུལ་བས་དགྱེས་ཤིང་ཚིམས།།
Lü kyi chö jin phul vei gyes shing tsim
By the generosity of offering the body, all are pleased and satisfied,

འགྲོ་ཀུན་སྡུག་བསྔལ་ཀུན་ལས་གྲོལ་བར་ཤོག།
Dro kün dug ngal kün le dröl war shog
May sentient beings be liberated from all suffering,

རང་སེམས་འཁྲུལ་བའི་སྒྲིབ་པའི་གཞན་དབང་ལས།།
Rang sem trul pai drib pai shen wang le
Our mind, under the power of illusion and obscuration,

ཀུན་བཏགས་གཉིས་སུ་སྣང་བའི་ཆོས་རྣམས་ཀུན།།

Kün tak nyi su nang wai chö nam kün
Phenomena are imputed as dualistic appearances,

གདོད་ནས་མི་དམིགས་སྤྲོས་བྲལ་ནམ་མཁའ་ལྟར།།

Dö ne mi mig trö dral nam kha tar
Primordially they are non-conceptual and unfabricated like the sky,

ཡོངས་གྲུབ་དེ་བཞིན་ཉིད་ཀྱི་དབྱིངས་སུ་ཨ།།

Yong drub de shin nyid kyi ying su Ah
In the sphere of ultimate Suchness - Ah!

The text translation is:

In the space in front of you is the guru King of Medicine
In an assembly with four guests
Our self consciousness emerges from the crown of our head
And is transformed into red Vajrayogini holding a curved knife and skull cap
She cuts open our skull with the curved knife
The skull is placed on a natural fireplace
Inside the skull, the body is chopped fine like mustard seeds
Fire and wind purified, it becomes an infinite ocean of nectar
Expansive as the sky, the offering is endless
Everything becomes the perfect desires of all guests
From the heart of Vajrayogini countless offering dakinis emanate
(they bring all offerings to all guests)

OM AH HUNG (repeat 101 times)

Three jewels and three roots, the guests of the universe
Offering with respect to accomplish two merits
Highest protectors, the knowledge guest
Offers to you, asking you to perform actions and transmit siddhis
Six realm sentient beings, the compassion guest
Give to you, pacify all sufferings and may they achieve happiness
Eight classes of spirits, the karmic guest
Offering to you, may they have peace and a compassionate mind
All the union guru's wisdom's
Illusory manifestation
Giving the body offering, all are happy and satisfied
May all sentient beings be liberated from suffering
Our mind is covered by illusionary ignorance

All dualistic phenomena exists only in name
All perfectly in the state of emptiness

The practice is as follows:

We visualize Yuthok as presented on the thangka in front of us in the blue space. He is surrounded by the four groups of guests located in the four directions. The four groups are:

> The first group consists of the enlightened beings like Buddhas, bodhisattvas and all enlightened beings. We can call them VIP guests; the Three Jewels and Three Roots, the guests of the universe. The reason for making this offering to them is to accomplish the two merits, normal merits and absolute merit, as well as to receive the ultimate blessing.

> The second group consists of the protectors and are called knowledge guests, all those enlightened protectors of medicine and nature, such as Shanglon Dorje Dudul and the nine protectors of the Yuthok Nyingthig. The reason for making this offering to them is to remove our obstacles and receive supreme siddhis.

> The third group consists of all sentient beings or six *loka* beings like humans, animals, spirits and so on. The reason for making this offering is to give them love, kindness and happiness.

> The fourth group are the eight classes presenting wrathful and dangerous spirits. The reason for making this offering is to give peace and harmony to all the spirits.

These are the guests we are offering our body to. Our consciousness comes out of our crown chakra and transforms into Vajrayogini in her red colour. Our body is lying dead on the floor. That means our Buddhahood is coming out and we are in our pure state.

Then our awakened consciousness in the form of Vajrayogini, takes a sword and cuts the skull off our body in front of us. The skull becomes like a bowl the size of the universe, and our body is inside of it and our mind chops our body into pieces. Spontaneous fire and wind appear by the power of the mantra *Om Ah Hung* and transform our body into nectar that is like the unlimited space.

Normally we don't trust ourselves and we never think we could offer ourselves to the universe, but if our mind transfers to a divine deity, then we can change the view of ourselves and we can use the self's perfect potentiality as an offering. This is the main reason why our mind becomes the Vajrayogini.

The nectar can take on any quality desired by the four groups of guests. For example, it can become medicine for beings suffering from sickness or it can be food for the starving. Thus the nectar transforms into whatever will satisfy and please the guests. We imagine ourselves as liquid nectar or light and offer what is required to all sentient beings. This is a very good visualization, an effective mental exercise and it's also useful for our mind balance.

Offering to the Enlightened Beings

The first group of enlightened beings are the Buddhas. The light and nectar of ourself is offered to all Buddhas, Bodhisattvas and all enlightened beings.

Some people like to offer special or precious objects to the Buddhas and enlightened beings, wishing to accumulate good merit. When making an offering, some people can feel guilty if they don't have precious objects to offer. Instead, we can make the best possible offering to the Buddha in a very easy, practical and honest way by offering the self; a body offering in the form of light, flowers, fruits, beautiful fragrances, good to look at, good to touch, the most beautiful music and so on. Whatever you think would be good, you can offer it.

If we know how to use our mind, we are never too poor to make an offering. Just open your heart as much as you can and offer all you can envisage to all enlightened beings. That is the best offering for them and in turn you will achieve whatever you desire from them.

Offering to the Medicine Protectors

The second group is the knowledgeable guests, all those enlightened protectors of medicine and nature.

There are several groups of Medicine protectors such as Rishis, Medicine Dakinis, Mamos and Tsomans, and other special protectors such as Medicine Mahakala, Shanglon Dorje Dudul, and still there are others who protect the practices of Traditional Tibetan Medicine and Yuthok Nyingthig.

In our offering to the protector, we have to offer a fluid called the 'Golden Drink' which can be liquids like alcohol, tea or milk. A solid offering is called a *Torma* which is a special ritual cake. We offer the most pure and infinite nectars and light and whatever else they need, such as a white offering, a red offering or *Torma* offering.

When I'm in Tibet, I try to offer tea, alcohol or milk to the protectors however when travelling it can be difficult and not always practical. Sometimes I couldn't offer anything and I felt bad about that. My life used to be busier making it more difficult to make the offerings. But when I started doing the Yuthok Nyingthig and really thinking of the meaning of the practice, I discovered that I had the ability to make an offering with me all along. The container is universal space and the perfect substance is my visualisation offerings.

One time, I was in Russia preparing for protector practice with a group of people. They wanted to use good quality alcohol but when I mentioned that they could just use pure water and visualise it as the 'Golden Drink', the leader of the group became quite angry and upset with me. He said "How you can offer just water to the protectors, they need Golden Drink, alcohol". I told him "If the protectors are enlightened beings, they won't only accept alcohol, they'll also drink water too! Really, water is more important and healthier than alcohol, so I really don't think that the protectors will get upset with our water offering." He then remarked "My Guru told me that we have to offer alcohol, water is not good enough." He was so nervous about offering water. This person believed that he was doing a truly authentic and powerful practice and that I was the one who was ignorant of the true secret spiritual path.

If the protectors are enlightened, then they need only our good intentions and mental visualizations. If there are spirits needing material objects such as alcohol and blood, then they are surely not the enlightened ones. The very best offering for enlightened protectors who have good, positive intentions and who are performing beneficial actions by helping others, is infinite nectar and light.

Offering to all Sentient Beings

The third offering is to all sentient beings or sixth *realm* beings like humans and animals.

If we eat meat, it means an animal has had to die for us and in doing this, we build up karmic debts to these animals. A person has to kill the animal to feed meat to somebody else. There's the process of the killing, suffering and dying, together with all the accompanying emotions with the end result being the animal is dead. Eventually, the meat is sold at the supermarket and served to somebody. The person who killed the animal, all the people involved in the preparation and sale of the meat as well as the person who bought and ate the meat, are all going to have a karmic debt to the animal.

We accumulate karmic debts to hundreds of thousands of animals and somehow we have to pay this debt back.

We should also take into consideration our burying customs such as burning corpses or putting them in coffins under and above the ground. Even in death we're not willing to share our body and participate in the natural cycle. In our lifetime, we've probably fed on thousands of animals, and yet we're not willing to let our body repay this by letting it return to nature. Because we have such a strong attachment to our self and our body, even after death we still wish that our corpse would be buried well. In Tibet, there is the tradition of sky burials. I like this approach not just because I am Tibetan, but because it a perfect natural cycle, repaying our body back to nature.

In a very simple and practical way, the *Kusali* practice helps us transform ourselves into nectar and in doing so, we're able to repay our karmic debts to the sentient beings who have died for us. As we can't offer our body physically, we do it mentally by performing visualizations. In this way, our offering can be sent out to countless beings.

The main practice is the transformation of our body into nectar or light and offering it to the four groups of guests.

This offering to the six realms or sentient beings is extremely important. To those who are hungry and thirsty, we offer food and drink, to those who are in pain we offer medicine, to those who are sad and unhappy we offer happiness, and to those who are in great fear we offer peace.

With this practice we can even offer nectars to nature; fresh wind, sunlight and pure water for all plants, and offer positive energy for the earth.

Consider the following and choose what you want to focus on:

- For physical and mental sicknesses and for people and animals in pain, we offer perfect medicine. For those dying and those dead, we offer to release them from suffering and pain.
- For beings enduring poverty and hunger, we offer perfect food and drink suited to their desires.
- For natural disasters, we offer to purify and rebalance the elements back to pure energy.
- For pollution of air and water, we offer an absolute light to cleanse and dissolve all impurities.
- For those beings who are generally suffering in life, we offer to eliminate the cause and effect of the suffering.
- For those living with fear, in war, fighting and in conflict, we offer to eliminate fear and generate security.
- For those lost and without guides or the homeless, we offer to create a perfect space for them.
- For those threatened with extinction such as wild animals, orang-utans, bees and so on, we offer vital survival energy and to restore their habitat.
- For those imprisoned and for caged animals, we offer freedom.
- For fish and animals that are farmed, we offer to release and free them from suffering.
- For those killing animals, for hunters and fishermen, we offer to eliminate fear and bad karma.

- For global climate problems, we offer to generate perfect solar and lunar energy.
- For cosmic energy troubles, we offer to provide the energy of the five pure elements to the universe.
- For negative karma of all beings, we offer to purify and cleanse.
- For individual's personal problems and long distance individual healing, we offer to resolve problems and to find mental peace.
- For all beings killed for food including vegetables and herbs, we offer love and compassion.
- For all life force, we offer gratitude.

Offering to the Spirits

The fourth group is the eight classes representing wrathful and dangerous spirits.

In both Tibetan Buddhism and Tibetan medicine traditions, we believe in the existence of spirits in nature. Nature spirits can become challenging to people, we can get sick, can lose balance or have mental problems, etc. However there are various methods we can use to block or reflect their negative energies and sometimes, if really necessary like if they attack us, we can attack back using really strong mantras and rituals.

The reality is that even though they are evil nature spirits, they have their own fears and sufferings. We can see this in people too. Some people are very powerful and nasty and they can harm others but if we look inside of them, there have many fears and suffering. Somehow because of their trauma, they harm others. There's a reason why they exist and why they create obstacles for us and, if we keep trying to fight with them, maybe the battle will never cease. Instead of fighting, if we offer ourselves to them, they might become calm and happy and then the conflict will end.

If we wish to be a good practitioner, we need to develop universal compassion and equanimity including towards the bad spirits. If we can offer to them the compassion they need, they can be satisfied and they won't harm others.

There are some nature spirits who are positive spirits however if we disturb them, they may create provocations for us. By mining minerals and metals from the earth, sucking oil, cutting trees, polluting the rivers, lakes, and oceans, and by creating air pollution, producing toxic products, building nuclear power stations, atomic weapons etc, all these things we humans have caused and so of course, it might be understood when the good nature spirits become reactive.

Our best solution is not to fight with them with rituals, we have to understand and help them. At the very least, we can offer nectars and warming light to help them feel great peace and happiness for all. We must understand that all those beings are the illusory manifestation of the union guru's wisdom. By making this whole body offering all beings will be happy and satisfied. May all sentient beings be liberated from sufferings; this is our main goal.

Our mind is blinded by illusionary ignorance resulting in us having a dualistic vision and sometimes, it might be caused by not being aware of the nature of truth. All these dualistic phenomena exist only in name, they are just labels. Primordially, nothing exists without fabrications and like the sky all phenomena exists perfectly in the state of emptiness.

For the practice, chant and reflect on prayers to the nature spirits. Keep your mind in 'space' or emptiness as much as possible.

From time to time, follow this practice when you can and it will help bring more happiness and satisfaction to you and others; other's happiness is the main source of our own happiness. Physically we can't help many beings as we're limited by this material dimension of existence. However mentally we are free and we can generate infinite energy and positive thoughts to all beings.

At the end of the practice, all dissolves into space or emptiness and rests in the state of absolute emptiness. There is no obligation to do this practice everyday, but it would be good if you try to. Otherwise, you practice maybe once a week.

Puja - Spiritual Group Practice

This practice should be done in the evenings or after the seven days of Ngöndro. The Tibetan word *Tsog* means a spiritual fest. The main purpose is to make a commune and appease positive energies and spirits and to purify all negative spiritual energies.

In order to make a proper Puja, you have to make some sort of material offering such as tea, wine or small piece of meat or food.

This short version is composed by great Tibetan yogi Jigmed Lingpa.

Ram Yam Kam

རཡཁ།

ༀཨཿཧཱུྃ།

Om Ah Hung

ཚོགས་རྫས་འདོད་ཡོན་ཡེ་ཤེས་རོལ་པའི་རྒྱན།།

Tsog dze dö yön ye she rol pe gyen

Tsog substances, the five sense pleasure, ornamented by wisdom,

ཚོགས་རྗེ་ཚོགས་བདག་རིགས་འཛིན་བླ་མ་དང་།།

Tsog je tsog dag rig dzin lama dang

Masters and lords of the tsog, knowledge-holder lamas,

གདན་གསུམ་དཀྱིལ་འཁོར་གནས་ཡུལ་ཉེར་བཞིའི་བདག།

Den sum kyil khor ne yül nyer shi dak

Masters of three seats and mandalas, the twenty-four pure realms,

དཔའ་བོ་མཁའ་འགྲོ་དམ་ཅན་ཆོས་སྐྱོང་རྣམས།།

Pa wo kha dro dam chen chö kyong nam

Dakas and dakinis, samaya-holding protectors,

འདིར་གཤེགས་ལོངས་སྤྱོད་ཚོགས་ཀྱི་མཆོད་པ་བཞེས།།

Dir sheg long chö tsog kyi chö pa she

Come here and enjoy the offerings of the ganapuja

འགལ་འཁྲུལ་ནོངས་དང་དམ་ཚིག་ཉམས་ཆག་བཤགས།།

Gal trül nong dang dam tsig nyam chag shag

I confess all confusions, mistakes and broken samaya,

ཕྱི་ནང་བར་ཆད་ཆོས་ཀྱི་དབྱིངས་སུ་སྒྲོལ།།

Chi nang bar che chö kyi ying su drol

All outer and inner obstacles are liberated into the Dharma,

ལྷག་གཏོར་བཞེས་ལ་འཕྲིན་ལས་འགྲུབ་པར་མཛོད།།

Lhag tor she la trin le drub par dzö

Please take the remainder torma and perform all activity.

The translation is as follow:

> Puja substances, the five sense objects are ornamented by wisdom
> Puja lord, puja owner, and enlightened gurus
> (Enlightened ones from) Dimension of three mandalas and from the
> 24 pure dimensions
> Dakas and dakinis, and protectors with samayas
> Come here and enjoy the offerings of the ganapuja
> To purify all mistakes and broken samayas
> Outer and inner obstacles eliminate them in a state of Bodhidharma
> Please take the rest of the offerings and do all actions
>
> Guru deva dakini gana chakra sarva puja
> u sha-ta ba-ling-ta kha kha kha hi kha hi

This practice is performed with others in a group on special days in accordance with the lunar calendar. *Gana Puja* is a Sanskrit word and in Tibetan it is called *Tsog* (*Tshogs mchod*). It means spiritual fest where you can meet with your Sangha and share the practice with them.

Many tantric texts mention offerings of meat, alcohol and *Tormas* for Puja. There is a lot of misunderstanding about this practice. Many practitioners believed that you must offer meat, alcohol, and that people should eat meat and drink alcohol.

For example in the nineteenth century, in Rebkong Ngakmang, there were many Ngakpas who used to drink lots of alcohol and eat a lot of meat as well. But when the head master questioned the practitioner's spiritual quality, he found not one of the Ngakpa was qualified in the compassion practice. He therefore decreed a very strict rule that they were not to practice Puja as, without having compassion, nobody is qualified to do these practices.

Today, it's very common to see Tantric groups gathering for a meat and alcohol party which they called *Tsog* practice. They seem to just chant some kind of mantras and meditations and then they start to eat and drink till they get drunk. I think this spoils the spiritual practice, nothing about it is authentic.

Someone who is highly qualified in Tantric practice like Padmasambava may be able to do these things but for a normal practitioner, it can be detrimental to practice in this way. Actually, it's quite logical. We follow spiritual practices for peace of mind and good health so if we eat too much meat and drink too much alcohol in the name of spiritual practices, that's a contradiction! Eating meat creates more aggression and sadness and can cause metabolic and cardiovascular illness, while excessive alcohol drinking can cause of liver and bile illnesses. Is that good spiritual practice?

For Ngöndro practitioners, you should not eat meat or drink alcohol. Instead, for the offering just use simple tea or milk.

The phrase "Puja substances, the five sense objects are ornamented by the wisdom" is really talking about mental offerings, i.e. the actual material offering is less important than the mental offering. In other words we don't need to offer real alcohol or meat, it can all be visualized mentally.

The *tsog* is a kind of meditation and it's very important to know the meaning and train the mind to cultivate compassion and positive intention in order to purifying sins. At the end of the practice, all dissolves into space or emptiness and rests in the state of absolute emptiness.

Dedication

Whenever we practice, we need to save our good intentions. We can save them through dedicating our practice and reciting the Mantra of Interdependence.

Imagine that our daily practice is like a pure drop of water and to save it, we drop it into the ocean. In so doing, that single drop will exist for as long as the ocean remains. In the same way, if we save our good and virtuous energy gained from our practice, it will remain in the universe forever - even when we die, the merits remain and can spontaneously help others. Thus, the final dedication is an essential part of the Yuthok Nyingthig.

དགེ་བ་འདི་ཡིས་མྱུར་དུ་བདག །

Ge wa di yi nyur du dag
By the merit, may we quickly

སྨན་རྒྱལ་གཡུ་ཐོག་འགྲུབ་གྱུར་ནས། །

Men gyal Yuthok drub gyur ne
Achieve the state of Yuthok, the King of Medicine,

འགྲོ་བ་གཅིག་ཀྱང་མ་ལུས་པ། །

Dro wa chik kyang ma lü pa
And through this, may all beings,

དེ་ཡི་ས་ལ་འགོད་པར་ཤོག །

De yi sa la gö par shog
Be placed on this level.

Text translation is:

From the virtue of this practice
May we achieve the Yuthok state, the King of Medicine
And may all sentient beings
Realise that state.

Mantra of Interdependence

Om ye Dharma
hetu pra-bhawa he-tun teshun
tathagato haya-wadet
teshun tsa yo niro-dha ewam wadi
maha sharmana so-ha

Translation of this mantra is:

Of those things that arise from a cause,
The Tathagata has told the cause,
And also what their cessation is
This is the doctrine of the great recluse.

At the end of the practice, all dissolves into space or emptiness and rests in the state of absolute emptiness.

Conclusion

Other Ngöndro practices end with the Guru Yoga practice but in the Yuthok Nyingthig Ngöndro tradition, the Yuthok Guru Yoga is performed after the seven days of the Ngöndro practice.

If one knows the essence of Guru Yoga, then the whole Ngöndro itself is perfect Yuthok Guru Yoga. With the Ngöndro, one is always connected with Yuthok, understanding the true nature of Yuthok and of one's self and the great union of all which is beyond time and space.

Yuthok Guru Yoga is not part of this practice and will be presented in the next level. For the Preliminary Practice, Karma Yoga follows the seven day Ngöndro practice.

PART 3   THE APPLICATION

The Routine Ngöndro

Karma Yoga

"Abandon evil doing
Practice virtue well
Tame your own mind
This is the Buddha's tradition"

Buddha

When we complete the practice of Uncommon Ngöndro, we move onto the Routine practice. This is an important part of the Yuthok Nyingthig that we can continue routinely throughout our life. Whenever we like, we can do something for other people, to help and to make them happier.

The Routine Ngöndro has six important points:

1. Support charities

    As much as possible support charity projects by offering physical support, donations or doing volunteer work. Help the poor and sick. If somebody is suffering from hunger or thirst such as those in third world countries, we should help them directly or donate to charity organizations. The amount you give is not important but what is vital is that you help somebody on a regular basis. I often give small donations to those who are really in need and especially, help those who are really sick as well as the dying.

2. Save lives, save patients or animals

    The onset of pain is a most difficult time for all beings and if we can offer help, it is of benefit for others and for ourselves. To helping the sick and dying animals is also very important, we may have different bodies but we all have life. It doesn't matter about size, colour, wealth or profession, all people live and breathe the same, and it is the same for animals as well. Even though animals don't necessarily have human intelligence, they still have a valuable life and it is just as precious as a human life. Once a month or in each season, do something to save animals, fish, cats, mice, earth worms etc.

3. Spread Buddha's or Yuthok's teachings

    Introduce others to teachings such as TTM and the Yuthok Nyingthig practice. Doing this helps people learn and understand that through the teachings, there exists a different way of thinking. Many people are not aware of the Buddha's teachings or philosophy and it can be beneficial if you help somebody discovers it. This is not about converting people's beliefs, we must always remember what the Buddha said, "Qualified monks and scholars, just as you check gold's quality, through burning, cutting and analysis, so check my teachings. If it's right for you then take it. Don't just take it as a gesture of respect."

4. Create clinics and centres

    Create places where people can be treated or helped. These centres become a vital place for connecting our energy, keeping people together as well as helping them.

5. Put karma into action

    It is not only important to do mental karma but to put karma into real action, to do things that can help in any way. In your free time, go to hospitals or aged care centres to help and support them. Doing a solitary retreat, sitting and visualising is a good way to practice however to actually help somebody is essential.

6. Act for the environment

    Do something for the environment or liberate animals. There are schemes that plant trees, clean the environment days and even walking instead of driving is beneficial for both the environment and yourself.

    Chadral Rinpoche, one of the main qualified Dzogchen practitioners, is a strict vegetarian and as such saves the lives of thousands of fish and animals - he is a perfect example of a great Karma master.

    In the Buddhist tradition, there are ten Negative Actions which are to be avoided, and they are divided into three groups; Physical, Verbal and Mental.

The three Physical negative actions are:

- Killing - to intentionally kill another being whether human or animal
- Taking - what is not given, taking by force, stealing or by trickery
- Sexual misconduct - can harm others and lead to conflicts and problems

There are four Verbal negative acts:

- Lying - can create trouble and harm others
- Sowing discord - cause conflict in groups, family and community
- Harsh words - speaking offensively to deliberately hurt another

- Worthless chatter - weakens or lessens positive energy and spreads negativity

The three Mental negative acts are:

- Covetousness - includes all desirous and acquisitive thoughts
- Malicious thoughts - thinking or wishing harm upon others, and dangerous ideas
- Incorrect or wrong view - such as not believing in positive karma, taking a view towards harming others, or views of eternalism and nihilism.

Karma Yoga is the practice of mindfulness in our life; it is simple and offers great virtue. Karma is action and we can call it "good action yoga." Yoga in Tibetan is called *Neljor* (*rnal 'byor*) and it means to obtain the reality and truth. People generalise that yoga is a type of body exercise however there are in fact three types of yoga:

1. Body Yoga (*lus kyi rnal 'byor*)

   Through exercising the body, we experience absolute truth of our body nature. This refers to physical yoga movement when we perform the movements correctly. By doing the easy yoga such as Karma yoga, you can achieve great physical work for yourself and also for the benefit of others.

2. Voice Yoga (*ngag gi rnal 'byor*)

   Using mantras, we can achieve the true nature of energy and mind. Using positive speech through psychological consultation and giving good advice, we can help others through the power of our voice, even by simply talking.

3. Mind Yoga (*yid kyi rnal 'byor*)

   Through meditation and visualization we can realize our ultimate potential by simply using the mind positively.

Body energy is used to perform good actions. Just being a vegetarian and fasting are examples of body virtue which can save lives and help to balance our energy. These things we can do in our normal day to day life, helping others, saving animals or just being vegetarians, even being semi-vegetarian is beneficial to generating good energy. Eating less animal meat is good karma yoga. Practicing Voice yoga energy brings peace. Offering mental support by maintaing a positive mind helps bring serenity to all.

Prostrations

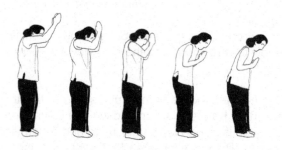

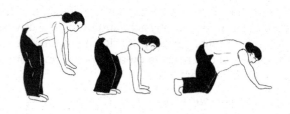

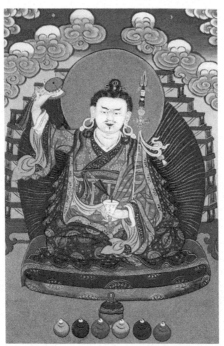

Dzogchen Choying Tobten Dorje

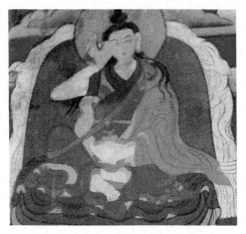

Shabkar Tsogdruk Rangdrol

རྣམ་སྣང་ཆོས་བདུན

Seven Meditation Postures of Vairocana

1 Sit crossed legged. Ideally in the full lotus position.

Balances descending ®.

2 Keep the spine straight, like a stack of golden coins.

Balances fire-accompanying ®.

3 Clasp the hands in vajra fists and press on the groins.

Balances descending ®.

4 Touch the tongue to the palate, just behind the teeth.

Balances life-sustaining ®.

5 Lift the shoulders up with straightened arms, like folded eagle's wings.

Balances all-pervading ®.

6 The chin should be slightly tucked in, like a swan.

Balances ascending ®.

7 Gaze at the tip of the nose, or into space just in front of it.

Balances life-sustaining ®.

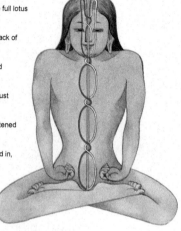

Right Channel རོ་མ (roma)	Central Channel དབུ་མ (uma)	Left Channel རྐྱང་མ (kyangma)
Anger/Hatred	Attachment/Desire	Ignorance/Delusion
Fire	Wind	Water and earth
Red	Blue	White
Solar	Neutral	Lunar
Bile	Wind	Phlegm
Snake	Rooster	Pig

© IATTM 2010

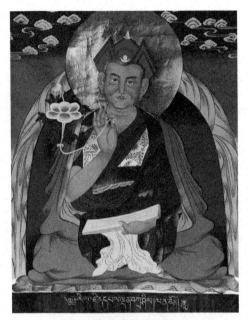

Rigzin Pelden Tashi

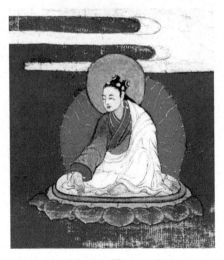

Yeshe Tsogyal

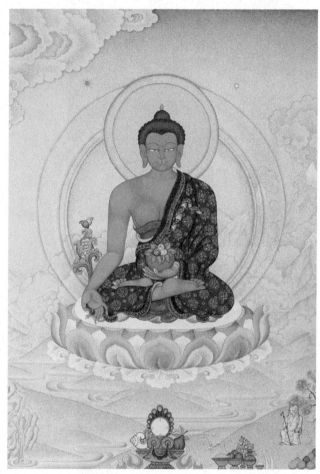

Medicine Buddha

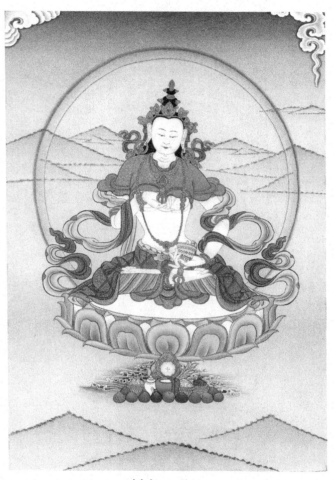

Vajrasattva

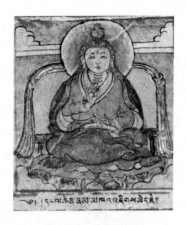

Changlung Pelchen
Namkha Jigmed

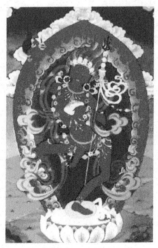

Varjayogini

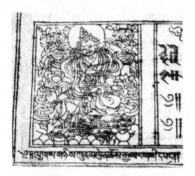

Chogyal Ngawang Dargye

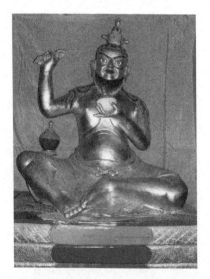

Khamla Namkha Gyatso

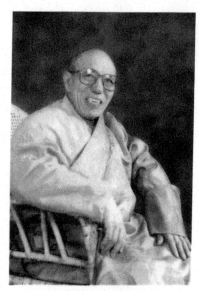

གཁཥད་བད་ཁྲོ་རུ་ཆོ་རྣམ།

Khenpo Troru Tsenam

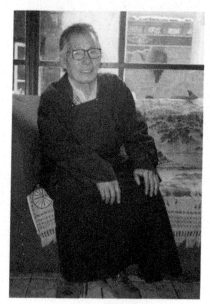

Chonyid Rinpoche

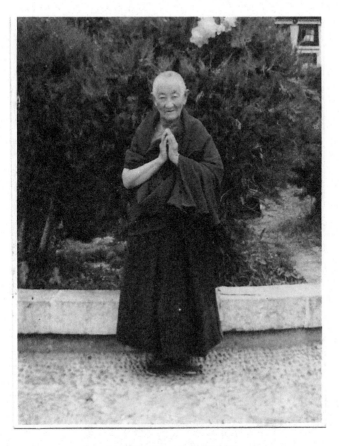

Ani Ngakwang Gyeltsen

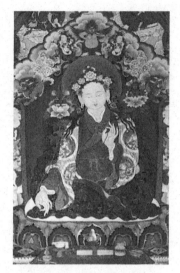

Yuthok -The Younger

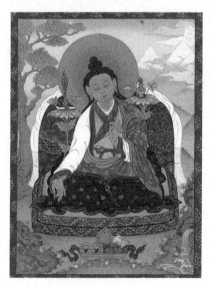

Yuthok -The Older

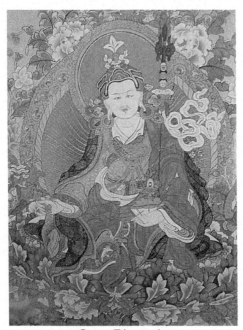

Guru Rinpoche
(Padmasambhava)

When thinking of the free style of Karma yoga, we should take any opportunity to help when it is presented such as:

- Helping patients
- Becoming involved in palliative care
- Supporting old people
- Offering to baby-sitting, to feed birds, stray cats and dogs
- Helping those people who live in difficult circumstances or who are homeless
- Volunteer wherever your energy can be of benefit

Karma Yoga is not only about doing physical work or volunteering in a spiritual centre, it's much more than that, any action with good motivation and a positive result is Karma Yoga.

With pure intention and positive motivation, everything can become perfect good karma.

Continue this practice as much as possible. Don't push yourself too much, just practice according to your life and when time permits. If you can practice only once a week or once a month it would be fine. What's important is to continue the practice and to keep the energy going because Ngöndro is an important foundation for Guru yoga.

This practice can bring you results where you will experience a happy mind, better quality of life, inner peace and joyfulness. Practicing Karma Yoga accumulates merit and wisdom for spiritual enlightenment.

PREPARATION

Positive Effects From the Practice

When doing the Yuthok Nyingthig practice, there are some particular signs that indicate that the practice is effective.

If your practice is performed mindfully and from the heart, you will meet Yuthok in person and he will guide your spiritual progress. If your practice is done with enough good intent, then you will meet Yuthok through visions and he will also guide you. And even if you practice in a simple way, you will meet Yuthok in a dream or will receive signs from a dream. As Yuthok's song says:

> *"Beseech me in a sincere way*
>
> *Overcome your lack of faith and*
>
> *Hope in me as if you give up your heart and mind to me*
>
> *A refuge throughout your life*
>
> *Immediately your two obscurations will diminish*
>
> *Upon meeting me in reality, in vision or in dream,*
>
> *I will reveal the path to the temporal and ultimate goal."*

Positive signs from the practice are:

- Feeling happiness; don't be alarmed if you feel sadness for the samsaric cycle of life. Should this happen, allow yourself to cry with compassion and devotion
- Enjoying the practice with a clear mind, feel balanced in mind, body and energy
- Not feeling tired or bored; finding solutions for problems; feeling energetic and positive motivation to help others; ability overcoming problems; feeling an intense freedom and happiness beyond all time and space
- Feeling great within the room or place where you're doing the practice and having a deep desire to stay in the retreat for a longer time

Positive dream signs:

- The dreams can have different meanings so it's important to remember them. You should write down your dreams every morning
- Signs of purification are dreams of having a shower, bathing, washing, cleaning, drinking clean water or tasty drinks, diving and swimming

- Dream signs of receiving good energy are a clear sky, sun shining, the moon rising, being in a nice place like a garden, a beautiful land, a forest or climbing mountains
- Signs that you are bring protected is when you dream of wild animals - wolves, eagles, bears or tigers - that they are kind towards you and you have a sense or feeling of being protected
- Signs of a healing power are saving fish or other animals, curing patients and helping others, finding herbs or working with plants
- Dream signs of Yuthok's body blessing are where you see or find Yuthok or Medicine Buddha statues or paintings, thangkas and other paintings or dream of meeting with holy people
- Signs of speech blessings are finding and reading medical or dharma texts, you hear pleasant music, songs, of speaking new languages or you have an extraordinary voice, or someone gives you good advice
- Signs of heart blessings are finding a stupa, crystals, gem stones or dreams where your mind is full of bliss, happiness and joy, even if you don't remember the dream you wake up feeling really happy and well
- Signs of Medicine Dakini and Medicine Rishi's blessings are seeing or meeting beautiful girls or unusual figures with healing powers, where they give you plants or flowers and teach you how to heal people and animals
- A special sign of eliminating negative karma is bad dreams or having difficulties in the dream, when our bad energy leaves from the mind and body. Sometime the process is difficult and this can appear as nightmares
- Good results of the practice are finding fruits and eating them, drinking delicious drinks, flying, reaching the top of a mountain or roof, crossing a river or lake, successfully accomplishing things in the dream, other people show respect to you, dreams about sitting on a throne or dressing nicely and being victorious
- Dreaming of meeting your master or holy people are blessings of knowledge, and finding gemstones or flowers are signs of healing empowerment

Sometimes Yuthok can manifest as a part of nature, as a light, rainbow, rain, wind or even manifest as an animal, and can teach you, support you or lead you in the correct or right directions in life.

Should you become ill or emotional when doing the practice, or your mind can't settle, then it's better to rest and try again another time. It's important you don't force yourself too much. Also, if you don't remember your dream, don't worry, it will come to you when you really need it to.

The Yuthok Mandala

The best place to prepare the mandala is in an isolated and quiet place or room, where there are no disturbances. Ensure you have enough food and drinks and anything you'd need for an emergency. If you can, arrange for someone to look after the cooking, that would be better than cooking yourself.

During the retreat, avoid meeting or talking with anyone who's not also doing the same retreat, and more importantly, if you're doing a solitary retreat, then you must not meet or talk to anybody.

The altar should be located in the east direction because Yuthok's practice is of peaceful action. It should be a one metre longer table covered by a white or yellow cloth. On the main wall, a blessed thangka of Yuthok should be hung, preferably on its own so that you only focus on Yuthok.

In the centre of the altar:

- Create a swastika symbol using rice and then cover it with a metal mandala which has been painted with saffron water
- On top of the mandala, place a card holder containing a small blessed Yuthok picture

In front of the mandala, there are should be all kinds of offerings, such as:

- Seven offering bowls of water
- Medicine offerings: golden Arura, camphor, sandalwood and six beneficial substances (cardamom, nutmeg, saffron, clove, long cardamom and bamboo pith)
- Fabric (only natural materials) in the five colours of blue, green, red, yellow and white
- Candles and gemstones, as many as possible

The below indicates the design of the altar.

YUTHOK ALTAR						
Gemstones	Medical Dharma texts	Mandala	Yuthok picture	Rice	Stupa	Five coloured fabrics
Offering water	Offering water	Offering water	Offering water	Offering water	Offering water	Offering water
Nutmeg	Saffron	Clove	Golden Arura	Cardamom	Long Cardamom	Bamboo Pith

What You Need for the Yuthok Retreat

The following is a concise list of items you need to prepare for the Yuthok Nyingthig retreat. You need to ensure you have all items before you begin the practice.

- Two sets of Mandala, one for the altar and one for self mandala offering
- White rice for the mandala
- Saffron threads for the water offering
- Card or picture holder and a small picture of Yuthok, the picture needs to be blessed
- Seven water bowls with saffron water
- Three fruits; Arura, Barura and Kyurura. The golden coloured Arura is the supreme choice for the practice
- Fabric made only of natural material in five basic colours; blue, green, red, yellow and white
- Candles and Gemstones, as many as you can gather
- Medicine offerings;
  - Six good substances of cardamom, nutmeg, saffron, clove, long cardamom and bamboo pith
  - Camphor
  - Sandalwood
- Fruit - any types
- Flowers - of various colours
- Incense - medical incense or Sorig incense
- A statue of Medicine Buddha for the circumambulations
- Alcohol for the *Tsog* offering and can be used in the offering bowl, if you wish
- A stupa or a picture of stupa
- A Tibetan Buddhist bell and dorje set for the practitioner
- Items to represent body, speech and mind such as a picture, text and a crystal
- For each participant in the retreat, provide a yoga mat. Light gloves are useful to protecting the hands when performing prostrations
- Offering herbs and spices which can be used for making medicine as well as for food

The Yuthok Practice Retreat

The Yuthok retreat can be carried out in a group setting or individually, i.e. on your own.

Yuthok Retreat on your own

The best location is an isolated or quiet place or room, being alone is best ensuring you will not be disturbed.

Make sure have enough food and drink and any emergency needs. Ask someone to cook for you if possible, otherwise its fine that you cook for yourself. During the retreat do not meet with anyone, there are to be no phone calls or internet contacts, only in an emergency.

Avoid reading other books, stories or watching TV because they can cause emotional and mental distractions. It's essential to just focus on the practice and to block all external contact. Traditionally, during the seven day practice, one typically follows a natural approach i.e. no bathing, no shaving or cutting the hair and no cleaning of the practice room. Food should be vegetarian, and certainly, there should be no consumption of alcohol, smoking (people should take this as an opportunity to quit!) or drugs. It's better to avoid drinks with caffeine and also be mindful that you don't eat or drink things that are too cold.

For the actual practice, you should complete four sessions per day, each session about two hours. Alternatively, do it twice per day, each session about three hours. By following these options, you'll be able to do 101 repetitions of each practice making it more practical.

Yuthok Retreat in a Group

The Yuthok Nyingthig course is presented in a residential setting. Traditional observances, such as a vegetarian diet are maintained throughout and the course is typically fully catered. Chanting will be in Tibetan phonetics.

Participants in this course must be committed to the practice of Tibetan medicine or healing. They will have studied previously with qualified doctors, or have done prior Tibetan medicine studies. Students should bring writing implements, a notebook, their own mala and a mandala set if they have one, and a yoga mat.

The Practice of the Protectors

Shanglon Dorje Dudul

ཤང་བློན་རྡོ་རྗེ་བདུད་འདུལ།

is known as The Medicine Mahakala, a Sanskrit word meaning protector of Dharma. In Tibetan,
he is Nagpo Chenpo.

མགོན་པོ་ནག་པོ་ཆེན་པོ།

He is the main guardian of the twelve protectors of the Medicine Buddha and was first mentioned in the Medicine Buddha Sutra, which gives clear indication that he is the supremely unique and perfect protector of the Medicine Buddha.

In Tibetan Vajrayana practice, he has three principal manifestations, outer, inner and secret. Commonly, the Medicine Mahakala is depicted in the form of the outer aspect where he is sitting on a lotus flower surrounded by five retinues including his consort.

According to the Yuthok Nyingthig Tradition, the outer aspect of Shanglon in the form of action is displayed riding a black horse surrounded by eight retinues.

Shanglon Dorje Dudul protects the Medicine Buddha, the Yuthok Nyingthig tradition and practitioners and of course, all those who pray to him. His eternal promise is that he will always guard and protect us and will fulfil our wishes in the relative aspect of life.

He is the enduring yet invisible wisdom guardian of our spiritual journey to enlightenment.

The Shanglon prayer

རཾ་ཡཾ་ཁཾ། ཨོཾ་ཨ་ཧཱུྃ། ཧ་ཧོ་ཧྲཱི།།
RAM YAM KHAM, OM A HUNG, HA HO HRI

སྨན་བསྲུང་ཞང་བློན་འཁོར་ལྔ་སྡེ་དགུ་ལ།།
Mensung Shanglon kornga degu la
Medicine Protector, Shanglon and his retinue,

གསོལ་བསྟོད་མཆོད་མགྲོན་རེ་བསྐོ་ཐུགས་དམ་བསྐང་།།
Soltod chodron re ngo tugtam kang
With praise and offerings, we invite you, may your heart be fulfilled.

ཕྱི་ནང་གསང་བའི་བར་ཆད་བཟློག་པ་དང་།།
Chi nang sangwai barche dokpa dang
Eliminate all inner, outer and secret obstacles.

ལས་བཞི་ལྷུན་འགྲུབ་མཆོག་ཐུན་དངོས་གྲུབ་སྩོལ།།

Leshi lhundrub choktun ngodrub tsol
And spontaneously accomplish the four actions,
transmit the Common and Uncommon Siddhis.

The Mantra is:

ཨོཾ་མ་ཧཱ་ཀཱ་ལ་ཡཀྴ་བཛྲ་ཙིཏྟ་ཧཱུྃ་ཕཊ་རཏྣ་སིདྡྷི་ཧཱུྃ།

OM MAHAKALA YAKSHA BEZAR (vajra) TSITA (citta)
HUNG PHET RATNA SIDDHI HUNG

Routine for the Yuthok Retreat

Before falling asleep, tell your mind that you want to remember your dreams. In your mind, pray to Yuthok in your own way asking him to tell or show you what you need to help you. If you have difficulty sleeping, drink fennel tea or make a soup with nutmeg and clove powder or even drink some warm milk.

In the morning, get up early and do the breath purification exercise, then go outside for some fresh air and maybe take a short walk as well. Eat a light breakfast, don't eat too heavily or too much. Before each meal, offer the food and drink to Yuthok.

When you go to the toilet, imagine that all bad energy is eliminating through the urine and stool. Should you sweat, picture that bad karma is leaving your body and when you have a shower, repeat the Dor-sem (Vajrasattva) mantra and visualisation. At all other free time, focus on the Dor-sem practice. If you take a walk, picture in your mind that you are doing circumambulation to the Medicine Buddha. Remember not to read other books, newspapers or watch TV; they can disrupt your mind. It's very important to be yourself and be connected with Yuthok all the time.

Most importantly, be mindful all the time and enjoy the practice; your every action is part of the practice and your every breath becomes virtue. Visualising this, you can devote and integrate all your energy, time and space to the practice.

Conclusion and Thanks

The Yuthok Nyingthig practice is a very ancient wisdom which has been passed from generation to generation. It is perfectly suitable and useful in our times; finally we have reached Yuthok's prophesied 'busy time'. From Yuthok's kindness, we are so fortunate to have this simple and wonderful practice, a foundation of spirituality as well as the essential practice of Buddha Dharma.

To follow this practice is like creating a small object; it takes only a week to finish but it is really important to do it with quality. The quantity and size is not important, to practice with your whole heart is the most important thing. This is first and basic practice and the final practice as well. Best wishes to you from my inner most heart.

> May this practice become a wisdom light for the beings who are in the darkness of ignorance.
>
> May this practice become an absolute nectar for the beings who are in the ocean of suffering.
>
> May this practice become a perfect medicine for the beings who are in countless sicknesses.
>
> May this practice bring infinite peace and happiness for all sentient beings and the universe.

I'm extremely grateful to all those who have helped and supported me in my journey of Tibetan medicine and spiritual practice, and especially those who've supported me in my professional field of Tibetan Medicine. Without their effort, I would not have stepped along this path on my own and most certainly, without my friends supporting me, the road would have been less enjoyable.

Ngak Mang Australia (and ATTM Australia) deserve special thanks for their effort and in particular in the production of this book. The Australian team have spent many hours working and re-editing this book. I always dreamed of setting up a publishing house and it was under their endeavour that the Sorig Publications came into being. I wish that under the Sorig Publications group, we will have huge success in publishing books on Tibetan medicine and healing arts.

My best wish is that everyone achieves immense happiness, peace and good karma in their lives, everyday.

Dr Nida Chenagtsang

APPENDICES

Appendix 1 – Questions and Answers

Please give further explanation about *gang ku sang chen ma*, the prayer to Yuthok

Yuthok's prayer expresses very deep concepts. Firstly, it refers to the fact that Yuthok's body represents the Sangha, his voice represents the Dharma, while the heart or mind of Yuthok depicts the Buddha. Another meaning of this prayer is the union of form and emptiness which is written in the Heart Sutra. This union is linked to the body of Yuthok, his voice is a unique fusion of sound and emptiness, while the heart or mind of Yuthok is the union of emptiness and supreme bliss.

Can you explain the symbolism of the representation of Yuthok?

In the thangka, Yuthok is dressed in a white robe which represents pacifying action. He sits in the lotus position indicating his achievement of realization, and his long black hair refers to wisdom. In this case, the color black refers to wisdom as it relates to the 'Protectors', who are usually black in color and are associated with spiritual guardians. The five flowers in his hair symbolize the five Dakinis.

In his right hand, he holds a blue Utpala flower that represents Tara, and on the flower there is a text and a sword which refer to the six *paramita* and to the wisdom of Manjushri, who is the Buddha of Wisdom. Therefore, Yuthok is both the manifestation of Tara and Manjushri. He manifests a great compassion and wisdom associated with perfect memory.

In his left hand he holds a pink lotus flower which means that he is an emanation of Avalokiteshvara, the Buddha of Compassion. This also affirms Yuthok's main practice of Dharma is to put compassion into action and for this reason he chose the medical profession. On the lotus flower, there is a Vajra which represents Vajrapani, the Buddha of Power.

In Tibetan culture we talk about *Rigsum Gonpo*, the three main Buddhas of which Yuthok is incarnate; Manjushri, Avalokitesvhara and Vajrapani.

Beside the Vajra, there is a pot or vase of nectar which represents the Medicine Buddha and indicates his ability to heal. On the vase, there sits a jewel which represents Ratnasambhava, the Buddha of Wealth, and finally an Arura flower which also symbolizes the Medicine Buddha, *Sangye Menla*.

Thus, the five symbols in Yuthok's left hand symbolize that Yuthok is the incarnation of the five Dhyani Buddhas, the five families, namely

Buddha, Karma, Padma, Ratna and Vajra. I want to reiterate that these symbols mean that Yuthok has all the capabilities of all the Buddhas.

The only thing that can change in the representation of Yuthok is the color of the aura that surrounds him. It is connected with the five elements and five actions; green - wind, wrath action; red - fire, control; white - water, peace; yellow - earth, growth; blue - space, all the actions.

All around Yuthok there is a rainbow which indicates that Yuthok achieved the great Rainbow Body or Light Body. In a text, Yuthok declared that he would communicate his presence through the rainbow and this is why he appears in this way. There are three levels of Rainbow Body; the smaller type or lower level is obtained when at the moment of death, the body shrinks. The second level can be recognized when the body is dissolved into the five elements but the impure parts like teeth, hair and nails remain. The great Rainbow Body is achieved when everything dissolves into space, including all impurities and clothes.

What does it mean to take refuge?

Normally, we consider that taking refuge in Buddha, Dharma and Sangha is the entrance into Buddhism, so in saying that when we take refuge, we become a Buddhist. However I believe that the true entrance to Buddhahood is not about taking refuge. There are verses of the Buddha that say "Students and monks, we cut and melt the gold to control its qualities. Similarly, you must analyze the quality of my teachings and decide whether they are suitable, then take them in a conscious way and not as a form of respect."

When you become a Buddhist, when you have full awareness of the teachings, you accept them deeply and assimilate them in everyway. It is known that the Buddha has always pointed out that he would not solve our problems but he would teach us how to solve them independently.

Who are the three jewels; the Buddha, Dharma and Sangha in which we take refuge during the practice of Bodhicitta?

The Buddha is the master, the Dharma is the teachings and the Sangha are the practitioners, and the three are referred to as the Supreme Jewels. In the context of Tibetan Medicine, the Sangha consists of enlightened beings; the Dharma is the teaching of Yuthok Nyingthig while the Buddha is the Medicine Buddha or Yuthok, which are all one.

The three jewels can further be explained in the following way; the supreme body of Yuthok is personified by the Sangha, the supreme voice of Yuthok is the Dharma and the Buddha is the heart or the mind of Yuthok.

Prayer is another way of taking refuge where the vows of the Bodhisattva are taken, which means practicing the Six Paramitas or the six perfections in order to attain a state of enlightenment, with the aim of helping sentient beings. It is therefore essential to practice the Six Paramitas with perfect intention because we accumulate merits to enable full realization.

Why is it important to do prostrations?

The blessing of Yuthok should be considered as pure nectar that we drink, but our container (our body and our mind) is impure and somehow, it inhibits the effects of the blessing itself. Therefore, purification occurs through prostrations.

Can you explain the mandala offering?

"The supreme and infinitely perfect" offering is the offer of the whole Universe to Yuthok and the more generously you make your offering, the more you receive in return from the Universe itself. The mandala offering does not need to be purified because it is already perfect. It is important to offer fully and generously, without limits.

Initially, in order to simplify the practice, we can offer what we ourselves really like. For example, if you like light, you can offer everything in the form of light, or for those who love flowers or jewelry you can imagine the offering in the form of such things.

How do you visualize the mandala offering?

The principle is to generate perfect generosity without attachment. When you offer the universe, you can visualize receiving the light that symbolizes the blessing of Yuthok to obtain wisdom and awareness.

During a retreat in France, a practitioner dreamt of giving the universe to a girl, yet hoped to receive something in return. The girl in the dream didn't give anything in return, disappointing the practitioner's expectations. As a result of the disappointment, the practitioner then dreamt of becoming a white bird locked in a cage. The girl in the dream then released him and he started to fly away, thus the practitioner received a very precious thing: freedom. He expected something physical, something material, but the gift can also be on emotional level.

Another simple way to visualize is to offer what we love most and in receiving the same. In any case it is important to remember that the offer is to be a perfect offering, beyond judgment.

It's useful to think of our breath; we emit carbon dioxide which is a poison for us but it is a source of life for plants. So we should not doubt the benefit of what we offer, but we must pay attention to the aim with which we make the offering because the more generously we offer, much more we receive. Be aware that the receiving however should not be our motivation.

There is also a Tibetan practice called *Tong len* in which we take in negativity and offer only positive things; this is a practice similar to the offering of the body.

Is there a difference between the short mantra and the extended mantra of Vajrasattva?

From an energetic point of view, the 100 syllable mantra is more powerful because of the higher vibrations that it produces. However, the most important aspect to the mantra is the visualization, through which the purification is generated. Therefore the short mantra, with good visualization, is effective.

Should we do all the visualizations mentioned in the practice of Kusali?

It is better for you to meditate on all the visualizations. Alternatively you can simply imagine that the body is transformed directly into nectar or light and then immediately offer it. It is important to understand the meaning of the offer which is to repay the karmic debt and cut the attachment to our body. Unlike what happens with mandala offerings, here we offer only our body which is transformed into nectar and then offered to the four different hosts. The reason why Vajrayogini cuts the crown skull is because it contains the brain and it is a symbol of our potential. We visualize that the crown skull becomes as large as the universe and in its interior is our body, this body is as big as the universe and it is transformed into nectar or light, indicating that our potential is endless.

Could you clarify further the Puja practice?

Traditionally, Puja is performed in approximately six to eight hours; this is a short version developed by Jigmed Lingpa (1729—1798) and introduced into the Yuthok Nyingthig around the Chakpori time i.e. when the Yuthok Nyingthig was a key practice of the University of Tibetan Medicine.

Gana Puja can be translated as a party with songs and dance, it is an essential practice to cleanse the internal and external obstacles (*ci nang bar ce*). The first of which relates to everyday problems such as work, personal relationships and family issues while the latter relates to mental and emotional problems. Also, a Puja is performed to repair the breaking of Samaya. Generally, we offer meat and alcohol and you can substitute meat with rice or barley, which is placed directly into the glass with alcohol. The offerings are divided into white offering, red offering and *torma*.

Offerings are first purified with *Ram Yam Kham* mantra which corresponds to the elements fire, wind and water, and then transformed into nectar through the mantra *Om A Hung*. Furthermore, the main point is the *Yeshe rol pe gyen* mentioned in the prayer, which means that substances are adorned by wisdom.

To better understand this concept there is a story about Yuthok, the elder. One day he was invited by his disciple who cooked meat. Yuthok said he was vegetarian and would not eat meat, but his pupil pointed out to him that it was Puja day and therefore the meat could be eaten. After some insistence, due to his reticence, the disciple asked him to use mantras to turn the meat in nectar; Yuthok did it but he still refused to take the nectar. He did this because he knew that many practitioners at that time confused Puja with the act of drinking alcohol and eating meat. If your ability is so high that you can turn meat into nectar, then to eat it or not is not important. The real offering is in fact created by the wisdom of the mind.

Who are the enlightened ones and the twenty four pure dimensions?

Enlightened beings of the three dimensions are the male Buddha, the female Buddha and the Buddha of the union of male and female. The twentyfour pure dimensions are related to twentyfour special places physically existing on earth but can be appreciated in the pure dimension only if we achieve the correct realization, i.e. when the gross wind dissolves through meditation into subtle wind, opening the doors of clear light and knowledge.

What does "left over offering" mean?

Lhag tor are the offerings that are left over. To understand this concept, we consider that in the pure dimension, there are totally enlightened beings and others that are only partially enlightened. For example, we first make our offerings to the highly enlightened beings, after which we then offer to the others such as the twentyeight Dakini with human bodies and animal heads.

What is emptiness?

Emptiness is a sophisticated, profound and essential concept of Buddhist philosophy. To simplify this view, we'll use a simple and practical example.

Usually when each practice ends (e.g. refuge, Bodhicitta etc.) there's a meditation about emptiness. An easy way of thinking about emptiness is to imagine that everything dissolves, including us, until there is nothing more. Through our practices, matter does not disappear but enables us to understand the true nature of phenomena; and we realize that which is written in the Heart Sutra, that "emptiness is form and form is emptiness". The experience of supreme emptiness is to see all things and, at the same time, understand their nature of emptiness. We see things and, at the same time, their atoms and particles of which they are composed are empty (all atoms are in fact 99% empty).

Therefore, we have to realize that emptiness does not mean empty, in the sense of lack of something or empty space, emptiness and fullness in fact coincide. Another thing to note is that illusory nature relates both to the subject and to the object, and realization of emptiness should cover us and the universe.

How should we meditate?

In general there are two types of meditation, an ordinary and an extraordinary one. The first is related to normal daily life and we realize spontaneously whenever we feel happiness and enjoyment. The purpose of many practices is in fact to make life more joyous, or achieve greater happiness, and through meditation we can pacify and balance our emotions.

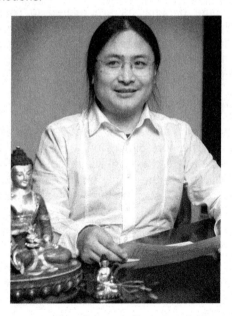

Extraordinary meditation is mostly associated with the unique spiritual path, which is deeply connected to the purpose of obtaining the highest achievement for the benefit of all beings.

How can I share this experience with others?

Normally there are secrets in spiritual teaching that can not be shared with people who have not received the initiation. The Yuthok Nyingthig Ngöndro however, can be exposed to people who do not follow the same spiritual path, in a similar way as the practices of Bodhicitta or The Four Immeasurables, for example, can be practiced by all.

We may practice yoga exercises, prostrations or meditate on the basic concepts of Tibetan Buddhist philosophy such as generosity; however it is of most importance that in all our practices, we do them with the clear intention of pursuing a path to enlightenment, for the benefit of all sentient beings.

It's not good however, to practice with people who have not received the teachings, but we can read them some text and discuss the contents with them.

When should we do the practice?

The practice of Ngöndro does not impose set requirements however it is preferable to carry out the complete practice in the morning, and at the evening to do Puja.

Each prayer may be repeated at least three times or more, depending on the time available. The practice can be done every day or whenever possible. The main thing is to understand with the mind and feel with the heart, for this reason it is not essential to recite the prayers in Tibetan, but it is essential to fully understand the practice and its meaning.

You should remember to put the practice into action. The practice should not just be in the form of words or thoughts but must always be transformed into action. In the Bodhicitta prayer we say: "with the merits obtained in practicing the six paramita". This prayer should not only be in the form of thoughts, but must be fully implemented.

Are there are specific practices to help all beings?

The Yuthok Nyingthig is a practice that develops a personal spiritual path and is useful in helping others too. Yuthok generated two treasures, two texts; the first, The Four Tantras, is designed to help people mainly in a physical way, through medical diagnosis and treatment.

The second treasure, the Yuthok Nyingthig, has a mainly spiritual nature. It helps to develop your spirituality including the balancing of energies. It helps an infinite number of beings through the practice of offering the body (purification) and healing, which you can not achieve in a physical dimension due to obvious limitations.

We need to always keep in mind that the energy of Yuthok is aimed at healing, as well as the Buddha of Medicine. Many teachers who have received visions of the Buddha of Medicine suggest that it's preferable to follow Yuthok's practice as he became incarnate as a human being and he is therefore better able to relate more to the human dimension.

Can we communicate directly with other sentient beings, or are our intentions only in the form of meditation?

To answer this question, I will tell you about a personal experience. It was when I was near Lake Baikal in Mongolia, where I had the same dream on two consecutive nights; the fish from the Lake asked me to help them. Upon awakening, I naturally did not know how to help the fish, and I really didn't know what would happen. After a few days, I walked right on Lake Baikal, which was completely frozen, and I saw a fisherman who was fishing from a hole in the ice. So, I went over and asked if I could free up some of his fish. Fortunately, the fisherman, who certainly thought that I was not completely sane, agreed to my request. So I took a fish and threw it into the hole, trying to return the fish back into the water. But the fish did not enter the hole and began to jiggle on the ice. I grabbed the fish, recited the mantra of Yuthok and, with a strong sense of compassion, blew the mantra over the head of the fish, then I put it in the water.

In the evening, while I was eating with my guests, the fisherman appeared. He was a very rich man who fished for sport, with no real need to fish for food. He turned to my friends telling them what had happened that morning, "A strange thing happened. After the Tibetan gave a kiss to a fish, I was no longer able to catch any fish". Somehow, my mantra freed the fish and at the same time announced a kind of warning which was broadcast to all the others.

This account is similar to another story about the famous Tibetan yogi Drugpa Kungle, who wrote a letter to the fish of the turquoise lake near Lhasa. At that time, in fact, there were fishermen who fished more than necessary and for this reason, Drugpa Kungle told them to stop fishing, but to no avail. So the yogi decided to apply directly to the fish, he wrote a letter to the fish and tossed it into the lake. From that moment on, the fishermen were no longer able to catch any fish.

These stories help us to understand that if our intentions are right and driven by compassion, we can achieve the most amazing things, and communicate with all sentient beings.

Can we do other practices and follow other traditions?

Of course you can follow other practices. Typically, there are two reasons why you decide to follow the teachings of Yuthok; the first is you decide that Yuthok Nyingthig is the main path to spiritual progress and the second is to create a connection with Yuthok. The later is called *drel jogpa* in Tibetan and means to create a connection or create a relationship.

What can we do to help the spirit of dead animals?

One of the best mantra is the Vajrasattva's mantra but also Avalokiteshvara's mantra (*om mane padme hung*) is very effective. These mantras can be recited in the presence of dead or dying animals or in the presence of animals in general.

Another very important aspect is to know how to behave in the presence of animals that are dying. Most often we're moved by compassion to kill them so as to avoid further suffering, but this actually blocks the purification process. Firstly, in euthanasia, we really don't know if the animal actually dies painlessly, and we think that to end the life process is part of Karmic action, which is purified completely. In fact, it is better not to interrupt the death process, but instead to pray with compassion from the heart, to alleviate all the suffering.

In this regard, I wish to share my own experience. Several years ago when I had already become a vegetarian, I was invited for lunch by my uncle. I accepted the invitation but I made him promise that he would not kill any animal - I knew about the custom of offering fresh meat for guests. However, when I arrived at my uncle's place, I realized that my uncle had killed a sheep to offer it as lunch. Of course I was angry with him, but he said that he killed the animal days before and that I should not think of it. Yet, it was evident to me that the animal was killed recently in line with my visit. This brought me pain, the animal had been sacrificed due to my presence as a sign of welcome.

So, with deep compassion, I started a practice to release the animal. After a while, I saw steam rising out from the plate of cooked meat and it formed the Tibetan letter 'A' which symbolized that the practice I had performed was effective and successful. Seeing this, it partly alleviated my sincere sorrow to the animal.

Should we be vegetarian?

Many teachers were vegetarian; like *Machig Ladron* the great tantric yogini who transmitted the practice of *Chod*; the great master *Ngagla Padma Dudul* who attained the rainbow body; the great Tibetan yogi *Nagkpa Shabkarpa Tsogdruk Rangdrol*. In his famous article published in a book "Compassion in Action", the teacher *Chadrel Rinpoche* stated that to be vegetarian and freeing animals are the best practices to achieve a long life.

There are however conflicting opinions. In his teachings, the great tantric master Padmasambhava mentioned two apparently conflicting concepts relating to eating meat. In one aspect, he affirms that "eating meat and drinking alcohol is part of the practice of Ganapuja", yet he then says "who eats meat has no compassion" which means that they don't have the foundation of spirituality. Because of their conflicting nature, these two concepts need to be carefully understood. You should only eat meat if you have real and high spiritual qualifications that enable you to release the animals, like the great master Tilopa did when he met his disciple Naropa for the first time.

Another thing to note is that in medicine, meat is considered a remedy for some diseases in which case you can eat it. It is only the need for a medical remedy that could justify the taking of meat or fish.

It is essential that you do not discriminate between large or small beings; they should all be considered in the same way, a life is a life, irrespective of the size of the animal. Importantly, to better understand the concept of compassion that lies at the heart of spirituality, when you follow a spiritual path or during a retreat, it is preferable to refrain from eating meat. In Chinese Buddhism, both monks and nuns are completely vegetarian, which I greatly appreciate.

Is it ok to take things from nature, like rocks, flowers and so on?

If you do, you should purify nature and space, so you should recite the Mantra of Interdependence.

Appendix 2 – Legends of the Rainbow Body

The Story of the Supreme Physician of the Himalayas

A biography of Yuthok Yonten Gonpo the Elder (729—854 AC), an extraordinary healing family.

In the seventh century, the most outstanding physician of the Tibetan King *Songtsen Gampo* was called *Lodro Shenyen*. In his family, Lodro was the lineage holder of Tibetan medicine and practiced Tibetan medicine for most of his life. His medical education was passed down from his ancestors.

With his beloved wife *Jomo Lodro Sangmo*, they had a child who also trained in Tibetan medicine, especially their family lineage of medicine; pulse reading, diet, herbal remedies, moxa and blood letting therapies. At a young age, he quickly became an extremely good doctor, continuing his studies of medicine with other masters as well. Because of his excellent medical wisdom, he was offered the position of the King's personal physician; and so became the personal physician of King Gungsong Gungtsan.

The son of Jomo & Lodro was the famous Tibetan healing doctor called *Dreje Gyagar Bazar*. The name Dreje was his title which means 'the master of spirits'; he was well-known for healing diseases caused by spirits or invisible beings. His home town was Todlung Kyidna which is a beautiful small village surrounded by farms and many high mountains near Lhasa, the capital city of Tibet. Dreje received many patients from all over Tibet as he was considered to be the best physician in Tibet in that time. He worked tirelessly, treating sick people without any interruptions and at times, he even visited invisible beings in other realms as well. Certainly, he taught his disciples both theory and practice, and his free time was dedicated mainly to spiritual practices.

One day Dreje went to check on one of his patients. When he reached the bridge of the Todlung River, a beautiful young girl came to him and asked him to visit her father. He said "Spirit girl, I'm busy with my patient. Don't disturb my work." She pleaded with him "Please great healer, you are the best healer for humans and spirits. My father is in a very bad condition and he needs urgent treatment. You who have such great compassion, you who treat all sentient beings equally, please help my father!"

"Where is your father now?" Dreje asked her. "He is in that high rock", she pointed to a large rock on the peak of the high mountain. "That is too far for today, I'll come tomorrow". Dreje thought, there isn't enough time today to climb that high mountain and the large rock. She continued "Don't worry, you can travel on my scarf" she said and immediately put the scarf on the floor.

When he stepped on the scarf, Dreje found himself already inside of the massive rock. There, he could see a very large hall and in the back, a big black man was lamenting, "Pain, pain!" Dreje asked him what happened to him. The big man said "I'm the local land spirit and I went to a place to storm their fields, but unfortunately there was a strong Ngakpa and he threw the master seed back at me. The seeds hit and wounded me" and the spirit opened his dress and showed his abdomen. Then Dreje said "I can cure you this time, but you'll have to promise me that you won't disturb the people's fields any more". The spirit said "I will promise you and I won't do any bad things in the future".

Dreje took the seeds out from his body and applied some herbal medicines. Immediately the spirit felt better. He was grateful for the healing and offered many precious things to Dreje. The girl took Dreje back and told him "I will bring some gifts. Please come to the bridge tomorrow". The next day Dreje went to the bridge but the girl did not appear. He thought it was unusual as normally, the spirits don't lie so he decided to wait for a while. Then he saw something being carried by the river and it stopped next to the bridge. When he went down to see what it was, it was a big bag of turquoise. He knew it was the gift from the spirit girl and took it home. Of course the bag was wet, so he put the big turquoise pieces on the roof of his house to dry.

When some of the local people saw that their doctor's roof was covered with turquoise, they began to call him doctor of The Turquoise Roof i.e. "Yuthok" (gYuthog). In Tibetan, 'Yu' means turquoise and 'thok' is roof.

Dreje continued to travel to many Himalayan regions for study and research. During his travels, he met human and non-human sages and learnt countless different ways of healing and about natural medicines. When he travelled to India, he met Nagarjuna's energy body and received many teachings on natural healing skills from him. Nagarjuna asked him to obtain more teachings from the Medicine Dakini (Lhamo Dudtsima) and the eight Dakinis.

So, he went everywhere in search for the Dakinis but could not find them. Then one day he went into the forest and there, he saw the Medicine Dakinis working on herbs. When he asked them for teachings they said "Do you have enough gold for these teachings?" He didn't and the Dakinis suggested that he go into the village and find some work. Yuthok thought that he could perhaps earn some gold in the village by offering his medical help to patients in the village. In the village, he met a young girl who asked him "Are you a doctor? Do you know about medicines?"

He said, "Yes, I'm a doctor from Tibet". "Then please come to cure my father, he is very ill at the moment and nobody can help him". So he went to their home and checked her father's condition, where he diagnosed and easily treated his condition. When the patient was cured, they were so happy and appreciative of his help that they offered a lot of gold. Dreje thought it was perfect, he could offer the gold to Dakinis and obtain the teaching. So, he travelled back into the forest where he met the Dakinis and immediately offered them the gold. Interestingly, the main Dakini then announced that they didn't really need the gold, that in fact, it was a lesson to show Yuthok the value and preciousness of the Dakini's teachings. It was important that he should have the correct appreciation of their teachings. Then she transmitted to him the *Dudtsi Mentreng* and the *Dudtsi Mendrub* practices. This is the complete medicine and spiritual union practice, which is so rarely received.

Dreje was overjoyed to receive all the Medicine Dakini teachings and wanted to transmit and preserve all those important teachings and wisdom in Tibet. Upon his returned home from his long studious journey, he decided to settle down in his home town and married Princess Gakyongma.

They had a son who was called *Yuthok Khyengpo Dorje*. At a young age he was seen to be very talented and learned all medical knowledge from his father, including the theory of the five elements, diagnostic methods, pulse reading and urine analysis, life style and diet, external therapies and methods for wound healing. When he performed his family's spiritual practice for medicine, he had a vision of the Medicine Dakinis and sages and from that he was blessed with a special healing power. This power enabled him to see a patient's body from head to toe and inside as well, as though they were made of clear glass. Ultimately, he worked and dedicated his whole life to treating and helping patients, donating medicines without any pride or bad intentions. He wrote the following for future Tibetan doctors:

King of Medicine, you are the supreme reincarnation (his father)
With your guidance I have learnt the general medicine
I have studied and gained the knowledge
By the deeper practice, I can see the real illness
With many patients I have gained the knowledge of practice
I'm not afraid of pain from disease
I can accomplish all patients' wishes
This is the gratitude of all Rigzins, Lamas and sages
Also the blessing of the compassion
I, Khyengpo Dorje, happy and calm
Can command the cold and hot imbalances
To cure without contradiction
Make diagnosis with pulse reading
Give diet that is the good base of health
Use remedies that work directly on the imbalance
Curing the external with moxa and blood letting

Healing wounds without surgery
I kindly work with patients without any pride
Tirelessly working with patients
Equally cure all patients
Cure patients without sectarian ideas
And without attachment give medicine to all
If I don't keep that promise, the Doctor is wrong
If I pretend and tell lies, the Doctor is wrong
If I'm lazy and take alcohol, is wrong Doctor
Pretending to know things, is wrong Doctor
Blind cure is wrong Doctor
Shouting without knowing anything, is wrong Doctor
Give advice without experiences, wrong Doctor
Mixing hot and cold, is wrong Doctor
Giving wrong cure, is wrong Doctor
Contradicting diet and life style, is wrong Doctor
Without knowing external therapy, is wrong Doctor
Contradicting word and practice, is wrong Doctor
If he likes alcohol, then wrong Doctor
If he likes sin, wrong Doctor
Like higher people and dislike lower people, wrong Doctor
Practice sexual misconduct, then wrong Doctor
Using wrong speech and causing problems, wrong Doctor
Don't know how to prepare formula, then wrong Doctor
Knowing much philosophy, is good Doctor
Knowing much oral teachings, is good Doctor
Knowing right words and meanings, then good Doctor
Using good antidote, then good Doctor
Precise practice is good Doctor
Having supreme compassion is good Doctor.

Dreje Bazar was happy and proud of his son's knowledge and skills. He prophesised that his son and their family lineage would continue for many generations and that they will develop and spread Tibetan medicine all over Tibet to benefit countless people.

Yuthok Khyengpo Dorje married Gyaza Chodon; they were a happy couple and were known as a beautiful family. One night his wife had a dream that a white man came to her and said "The Medicine Buddha is inside you, please keep him well". On that day, she received a sign that she was pregnant.

On the tenth day of the Monkey month in the Monkey year, a very strong light radiated from the east and entered into her heart. Then, many medicine Dakinis, protectors and sages came to her and said that the Medicine Buddha would be born soon.

On the fifteenth day of the Monkey month, the greatest Tibetan physician was born early in the morning. Colourful rainbows appeared in the sky, lights and music naturally and spontaneously appeared. In the Tibetan culture, this is a magnificent sign of the birth of a great reincarnation of a Bodhisattva. The baby was born very easily, without any obstacles and the delivery was pleasant. Everyone was very happy. His parents called him Yonten Gonpo meaning the Lord of Knowledge, and they hoped that he would become a great physician with the full knowledge of Traditional Tibetan Medicine, to carry on their family lineage.

Yuthok's childhood

Yonten Gonpo was a happy, calm baby and his parent's found him pleasant and easy to take care of. One day, at the age of three, he declared to his mother "I feel pity and compassion." His mother asked "For who?" to which his reply was "For all patients (who are suffering with illness)".

On another occasion, he said to his mother "Look into space". His mother said "Who is there? I can't see anybody." Yonten said "I can see Medicine Buddha, Medicine sages and Medicine Dakinis." It was then that his mother became aware that her son Yonten was receiving visions of the Medicine Buddha and other beings.

When Yonten was five years old, his mother had a dream that Mahakala told her that Yonten should receive the teaching of *Dudtsi Mendrub*, a spiritual practice of medicine. When she told her husband about it, he knew her dream was a sign that he should now pass on the family lineage teachings to his son and so, he shared the transmission of the family's practices with his son. From that time on, Yuthok Yonten Gonpo gained a vast knowledge and his medical practice advanced extensively.

Five years later, the King of Mei Ag Tsom invited him to the Samye Palace. There, Yuthok's medical expertise was tested against many other older Tibetan doctors. Without fault, Yuthok showed his exceptional understanding of Traditional Tibetan Medicine such that the King offered him the position of head doctor.

At the Palace, Yuthok was asked to cure many difficult cases of patients. A paralysed person came to Yuthok requesting a cure. After checking the patient's pulse, Yuthok said that what he needed was stretching and he offered to stretch out the patient using the King's horse. When the patient heard this, he jumped up and ran away. Everybody was shocked by Yuthok's accurate cure. When the King asked him about the patient's cure, Yuthok replied "The patient was not moving about and so his muscles were stiff. This was causing breathing problems and paralysis for the patient, so I got the man to stretch his muscles and now his lungs are fine."

The King was very surprised and he offered his horse as a gift to Yuthok. When Yuthok returned home, he gave the horse to his parents.

By the age of fifteen, the King Trisong Detsan invited Yuthok to his palace to cure his eye problems. When Yuthok went to the King, he explained "There's a bigger problem here, if you're not careful, you might develop a toxic growth." This worried the King and he asked Yuthok how to prevent it. Yuthok suggested that he practice a special massage every day. The King followed the massage as he was instructed and, as he thought his fingers were not clean he didn't touch his eyes, thus his eye problem was cured.

While he was in Samye, Yuthok visited a famous *Ngakmo* who was called Tokpai Randrol. She greeted him saying "You are the emanation of the Medicine Buddha and all people who have connection with you will be reborn in the realm of the Medicine Buddha." She then asked to know about Yuthok's spiritual experience. After hearing about his experiences, she was delighted and offered to share the transmission of the Dakini's practice with Yuthok.

At the age of twenty, Yuthok had a long and intensive debate with nine qualified doctors from all over Asia and a Chinese doctor questioned him about the history of Tibetan medicine. Yuthok explained that since the period of King Kha Thothori Nyantsan there had been a strong tradition of Tibetan medicine and it had continued until this time.

Further Studies in Asian Countries

One day, at the age of twentyfive, Yuthok had a vision of a young girl who proclaimed "Dr Yuthok, you should go to India." Even though the King wanted him to remain in Tibet, Yuthok decided to visit India to learn more about medicine.

Before his first journey to India, Yuthok went to meet the great Guru Padmasambava, to receive teachings from him, a mantra protection and a medicine protection. On his journey, he met the Nepalese doctor Bhanashilaha who invited Yuthok to Nepal, which he accepted. Yuthok stayed with the doctor in Nepal for several months and in that time, he visited many patients and studied Nepalese Medicines. He also met the famous Tibetan translator Berotsana who advised him to study medicine with Chandra Deva.

By the time Yuthok returned to Tibet, he had acquired a great deal of new knowledge as he had studied in India for three years and also spent time in Nepal on the way. Upon his return, the Tibetan King was really happy to see him and celebrated his return. Back home, Yuthok used and applied his newly developed skills on his patients with excellent results.

When Yuthok was thirtyfive years old, a white man came to him in his dreams and announced "Yuthok, go to India". He knew then that this was his second chance to go to India which he embraced. This time in India, he met with one hundred and one Indian physicians and scholars; he studied and exchanged his knowledge with all of them, which greatly deepened his knowledge.

When he eventually returned to Tibet again, he proceeded to share his knowledge with nine other scholars. His teaching method included having his students study general medicine during the day and Dharma teachings at night. Yuthok also gave them a very detailed explanation on the Arura tree. Once, in the presence of his students, he performed the very first mercury purification (detoxification) practice using substances and mantras. Around that time, the Khache King was ill with gout and Yuthok offered to treat him, prescibing that he take some mercury pills. After taking the medicine, the King was completely cured and was so delighted that he offered Yuthok gifts of magnificent pearls and other gemstones. Following the success of this treatment, Yuthok was inspired to offer an extensive teaching on the mercury medicine.

After that, Yuthok travelled to Drak Yerpa to follow a five day retreat in Padmasambava's cave. During this retreat, he had a vision of Lhamo Dudtsima who told him that his family lineage would continue and that there would be another Yuthok. She also described his disciples and family lineage; past and future.

Some of his students asked Yuthok about his family medical spiritual practice; he told them that this medicine empowerment could actually prolong a person's life. Yuthok explained that there existed three types of life a person could experience; a long life of 120 years, a medium life of 90 years and a short life of only 10 years. He taught them about the practice of Pulse Meditation with the eight Medicine Dakinis and three Sages. For this practice, it's very important to follow primary practices such as Medicine Blessing and Mind Introductions etc, and Yuthok gave these teachings to his disciples, telling them to practice them thoroughly. Furthermore, he gave them permission to spread his teachings to other people in the future.

One day, the Nepalese King became quite ill so he invited Yuthok to visit Nepal to cure him. Yuthok journeyed to Nepal with his people where they met with the Nepalese physician Shrisnaha. Yuthok consulted the King, checking his pulse, and advised the King that he had a cold condition. Shrisnaha disagreed, saying his condition was instead hot, not cold and suggested the King should avoid the four poisons, sun light - the poison of skin, salt - the poison of bones, alcohol – the poison of muscles and sex - the poison of body.

But Yuthok said that if the King avoided them completely, he would just become more imbalanced, and recounted the story of a Yogi who decided to avoid those same four poisons only to then become very ill. The Bodhisattva Tara came to the Yogi and instructed him to make use of those four poisons, after which the man was cured.

Shrisnaha said "I don't believe you" so they consulted a famous Nepalese sage asking him which one of them was right. The sage said Yuthok was right. The King then followed Yuthok's instructions, and was cured by Yuthok's treatment. Shrisnaha was surprised by Yuthok's healing knowledge and decided to commence studying with Yuthok. Later on, after studying successfully with Yuthok, the local people referred to Shrisnaha as the second Yuthok, the Yuthok of Nepal.

When Yuthok reached thirtyeight, he travelled to India for the third time staying there for four years. On the way to India however, Yuthok stopped in Nepal for six months, where he received teachings in tantric studies and Dzogchen from Parbahati Mahamudra. Later on in India, he received a vision of the Medicine Buddha's pure land and received teachings from him.

In a non-Buddhist village, a Hindu master asked him which religion he followed and Yuthok replied that he took refuge in the Buddha Dharma. The villagers were incensed by this and took hold of Yuthok, throwing him into a toxic lake; Yuthok however transformed the lake into fire. They then burned him in a sandalwood fire, but Yuthok transformed it into water. Finally, the villagers attacked him with many weapons, but Yuthok transformed them into flowers. When the Hindu master challenged Yuthok to a debate, Yuthok won the debate. When he sent a paper horse, Yuthok visualized fire and burned it. At last, the Hindu master transformed himself into a bird and flew away, but Yuthok transformed into an eagle and chased him. The Hindu master quickly transformed into a fish, but Yuthok transformed into a fisherman and caught him. Finally, the Hindu master did not know what else to do, so he decided to become a Buddhist.

During his stay in India, Yuthok met and studied with the master Mewang, learning many special medicine texts and techniques from him. Yuthok also studied at the Nalanda Monastery and he met and studied with the master Shungche from who he received teachings in Astrology and Astronomy. When he finally returned to Tibet, all his disciples and patients rejoiced in his return.

The First Tibetan Medicine Centre in Menlung

The King Trisong Detsan offered the place of Kongpo to Yuthok to allow him the opportunity to develop his medicine projects. Kongpo is located in the east of central Tibet and is well known for having a very good climate and natural medicine resources such as wild plants, flowers, minerals and salts as well as many wild animals. Yuthok took up residence in a place called Menlung, which is a small area in Kongpo.

At fortytwo years of age, Yuthok entered into a three week retreat in Menlung and on the fifteenth day, he saw a great white light and inside the light there appeared the Medicine Buddha surrounded by many other Buddhas. In this vision, the Medicine Buddha gave Yuthok further teachings and prophecies. In Menlung, Yuthok continued to treat many patients who came to him whilst still maintaining his tradition of daytime teaching and night time meditation.

One day a girl came to him offering some gemstones and asking him to visit her sister. Yuthok asked the girl "Who are you?" to which she replied "I am a Naga girl and my sister is sick, please come to our home." Yuthok said "I can't cure Nagas" but the girl insisted "Just like your grandfather, you can cure all beings. Please come and cure our sister." "How can I get there?" Yuthok asked her. The girl showed him a mirror and through the mirror, they were immediately transported to the Naga realm. There Yuthok saw a beautiful girl who was very sick and immediately he knew the cause of her illness; people had polluted the water causing illness to the Nagas. He gave her a shower with saffron water, administered some medicines and then performed some special rituals. After Yuthok's treatment, the Naga girl was cured. In gratitude, she offered Yuthok a special turquoise umbrella and her sister offered him a vajra and mirror as well as many precious jewels.

When Yuthok returned to the human realm, he often used the turquoise umbrella and thus became known as 'Yuthok with the turquoise umbrella'. As a result of curing the Naga, he became especially famous and many patients and students came to see him. He also wrote many texts on Medicine and taught people about his new knowledge.

At the age of fortyeight, Yuthok completed the 'Four Medical Tantra' (rGyud-bZhi) text and wrote many other texts using them as educational or teaching texts for his disciples. By the time he reached fifty, Yuthok had three hundred disciples which he taught the 'Four Medical Tantra' teachings and of most importance, he established a medical educational system very similar to the current system taught in universities today. Under Yuthok's system, a student studying the equivalent of a PhD would have to complete the Four Medical Tantra, Somaradza (one of the oldest Tibetan medicine texts), Dudtsi Bhumpa (a gter-ma text called The Vase of Nectar), the Eight Branches with its Commentary and the Sage's Oral Transmission. For a Master's Degree, they would need to study the Four Medical Tantra, the full text of the nine Tibetan physicians, Somaradza and Dudtsi Bhumpa. For a General Practitioner, their curriculum would include the Four Medical Tantra i.e the Root Tantra, the Explanatory Tantra, Tantra of Oral Instruction and the Final Tantra.

This system of teaching medicine still exists in Tibet today. Yuthok founded the Tanadug Medicine School in Kongpo Menlung, where he had 1,000 disciples. Yuthok also received an invitation from the Chinese King who invited him to visit China. Yuthok did, curing many sick people including the Chinese King himself.

One day, Yuthok was doing a Dudtsi medicine practice and a girl came to him in a vision, advising him to go to Odiyana. Yuthok took heed and went at once and there he met the great Guru Padmasambhava. Around that time, as Yuthok travelled three times to India and once to Odiyana, people thought that he must be a Bodhisattva. When they went to examine him, Yuthok knew they'd come to observe him and his body transformed into a rainbow. When his people couldn't find him, they thought he might have died and his body carried away. Yuthok then showed his body and told them "Now my body is just like a light or a rainbow, there is no difference."

Soon after this, in the place called Kongpo, Yuthok built the first Tibetan medicine Centre for education and it was called Menlung Gonpa Tanadug. Yuthok taught there every day.

Marriage of the Rainbow Body Doctor

One night, Yuthok had a vision that a red man came to tell him to do a retreat for six months in a specific cave in Amdo. Initially it was difficult to locate the cave but Yuthok eventually found it in the snow covered Lachi Mountain where he performed gtummo practice for three weeks, causing all the snow to melt away around him. He remained in the cave in meditation for three years and three months. He encountered many wild animals and wolves approached as close as a domestic dogs, but with the care of his protectors, Yuthok was always kept safe from any danger. Finding the cave and doing the retreat was the foretold auspicious sign which indicated Yuthok's teachings would spread throughout the Amdo region.

When he finished the retreat, Yuthok visited his home town of Todlungkyina and the townsfolk were so pleased to see him, they offered him a lot of food. Yuthok said "I don't eat meat and I don't drink alcohol". This was the first time he gave teachings on Gana Puja saying that without the base of a really stable meditation practice, nobody should eat meat or drink alcohol.

Many of his disciples and patients had direct contact with Yuthok and thus asked him many questions, which Yuthok kindly and precisely answered. Yuthok especially focused on giving advice to his students in their spiritual practices.

Later, Yuthok returned to his medicine land Kongpo Menlong and again, all the people from that region were delighted to see him. Where ever Yuthok travelled, people were always happy to see him and genuinely welcomed him with all their hearts.

When Yuthok went on a long retreat at Yasang Mountain, he had a vision of Rahula who offered him the method and treatment of Rahu provocation. Additionally, Rahu promised that he would always protect Yuthok's teachings. Following that, Yuthok then went on a pilgrimage to Lhasa where he accomplished 100,000 circumambulation of Chokhang.

When he returned to Kongpo, Yuthok received a transmission from a Dakini for the treatment of mad dogs, but in order to receive this teaching, Yuthok had to display exceptional capacity. For example, he was thrown into a raging river; he was buried underground; burned; cut with a sword and thrown from steep rocks. Yet his illusory body was not affected by any of these external attacks, so the Dakini learned that Yuthok was a highly realized Rainbow Body Master, the state of Light Body.

At the ripe age of eightyfive, Yuthok married Dorje Tsomo and they had three sons.

Then Yuthok travelled to Ngari in West Tibet with 250 people and treated many people using medicines, mantras, visualizations, etc. In that region, there was a good physician called Thuchen, who was so jealous of Yuthok, he had one of his disciples to go to quiz Yuthok about his knowledge. So the disciple went to meet Yuthok and asked him many questions, which Yuthok answered willingly and precisely. The disciple was so surprised by Yuthok's wisdom, he decided to follow Yuthok. But when his teacher Thuchen discovered this, he was most unhappy that he'd lost his disciple to Yuthok that he carried out black magic against him. Yuthok calmed the disciple saying "Don't worry about black magic, all is illusion and like a dream. If you remember this well, black magic won't affect you." But the students were still a little unsettled and wanted to do something so Yuthok taught them how to do some protection rituals to protect from magic attacks, and they were never affected from the attack.

Yuthok went to the Sacha area where he meditated at the Manjushri cave and gave teachings to Kongchok Gyantsen about the behaviour of Tibetan doctors, instructing that it is essential to work with compassion. Yuthok journeyed to China with his disciples on a pilgrimage to Wuthai Mountain where he studied and researched Chinese herbs and therapies. One day, due to heavy rain and snow, he became lost and no one could find him, however Yuthok had found his way to a cave. In the cave, Yuthok had a vision of Tara who gave him a teaching of Medicine Dharma.

When Yuthok returned back from China, he met a lady who was a Ngakmo from Chayul, her name was Damey Mentsun. She said her father has passed away when she was five years of age and he had been a doctor. She had studied some medicine with her father and was good at studying. She asked Yuthok to teach her the rGyud-bZhi, the Four Tantra. Yuthok explained that there weren't many women studying Tibetan medicine and instructed her that, in order to become a good doctor like her father, she would have to study Tibetan medicine wholeheartedly and would need to always keep compassion and wisdom foremost in her life. That is important for all doctors. She followed Yuthok's teaching with fervour and then asked for spiritual teaching. Yuthok taught her the Medicine Dakini practice which she was to practice every morning to avoid laziness and desire and to have positive intention. She dedicated herself for a long time, working and studying very hard, becoming the most important female disciple of Yuthok.

Yuthok and some of his disciples went to Dagpo and while there, he gave teachings about diagnosis. He saw many hunters, fishermen, robbers and thieves and Yuthok felt very sad for them, so he prayed to Medicine Buddha asking that the people stop killing animals.

When he returned to his land, he gave the Medicine transmission to his three sons. He then went on a personal meditation retreat and he visited Nirvana with his wife Dorje Tsomo; his children and disciples were surprised by his journey to Nirvana. Through his spiritual practices, Yuthok voyaged to the pure land of the Medicine Buddha and received Medicine and teachings from the Medicine Buddha himself. He and his wife went to Odiyana where they met Guru Padmasambhava. One day, Yuthok gave many teachings and advice to his disciples and then travelled to the Tsang area for a pilgrimage. It was there where he gave spiritual teachings and offered advice to doctors. Then Yuthok went for a pilgrimage to Mount Kailash and on the way, he cured many sick people. He also went to Nepal where he taught and also cured many people.

At the age of 100, he taught the Medicine Dakini teachings. When he was 110 years old, while giving a Dudtsi Mendrub empowerment, the Torma melted in light and became very tasty. Then, it became full of light from space and Yuthok invited all the Buddhas, Medicine Sages, Dakinis and all people to witness this with their own eyes. One day, his student Palden Lhundrub asked Yuthok how many books he had written, Yuthok told him that he'd written about thirty books on Medicine, Astrology and spiritual practices. To this student, he gave a teaching on the Mind according to Rigpai Ralkor Nga.

When Yuthok was 120, he wrote the final medical book called Nyamtig Thongba Dontan and gave his final teaching to his disciples.

He told them that he would soon go to the Medicine Buddha's pure land where he would continue his activities.

In the Rat year, on the fifteenth day of the Monkey month, the great Yuthok achieved complete Rainbow Body with his wife Dorje Tsomo and their dog as well. Their bodies dissolved into light and rainbows, natural sounds were heard, the earth moved, five coloured lights were seen, a clear sky was experienced and it rained flowers for three months; all these are the signs of the highest realization.

Their three sons and their disciples built a liberation Stupa and statues of Buddhas in memory of Yuthok.

Yuthok Yonten Gonpo the Younger - A Great Rainbow Body Physician

As a three year old child he used to behave as a doctor when amongst other children, feeling their pulse and examining their urine, and recognize herbs and minerals used in pharmacology. At the age of eight he began to study Tibetan medicine with his father and from other teachers, he learnt about Buddhism, arts and languages; he became exceptionally learned in everything he studied.

When he was fourteen, one night he dreamt of a deity called Drupa'i Lhamo who came to him dressed in blue and holding a vase filled with nectar. "The Medicine Buddha" she said "told me to bring you this vase filled with nectar. Please drink the nectar". When the boy drank the nectar, his body became pure and limpid like crystal. Then she made the following prophecy "In two years from now, you will encounter the Four Tantras of Medicine. These tantras will enable you to accomplish the benefit of many beings." Awakening from that dream, he felt extremely happy.

This boy was to become one of the most famous Tibetan doctors and masters, Yuthok Yonten Gonpo. He was born in the village of Goshi Rethang in Western Tibet, on the eighth lunar day of the last summer month of the year 1126. His father was Khyungpo Dorje and his mother Pema Oden.

The day after Yuthok had the dream, a Geshe called Roton came to him and asked to be treated for a severe case of rheumatism in his legs. Yuthok treated him successfully. Later, Roton went to Central Tibet and stayed for two years, where he contracted a malignant disease, trying different treatments which failed to cure him. It was only with the help of Upa Dardrak, a renowned doctor from Central Tibet, that the problem was resolved. Roton came to learn that Upa had the transmission of the Four Tantras of Medicine and studied all the Four Tantras and their commentaries with him. From Upa, Roton received the three traditions of the practice of the Medicine Goddess and the permission for the practice of Nochin Shanglon, the special guardian of Tibetan medicine and doctors. When Roton returned to Western Tibet, he believed that if he transmitted the Four Tantras to Yuthok, Yuthok would be able to preserve and propagate the teachings. Roton and Yuthok discussed the content of the Four Tantras and they identified medical knowledge not covered in them. Roton showed a remarkable knowledge which convinced Yuthok to study the Four Tantras with him. For a while, Yuthok kept the knowledge of the Four Tantras to himself and did not teach them to others.

At the age of eighteen he travelled to India for the first time. In a place called Kuda'i Ling, he met the Dakini Mandarava who gave him the transmission of the Cahnglo Ngakpo Tantra. Then he proceeded to Varanasi where he studied the Eight Branches of Healing, the Somaradza, and other treatises on Medicine. On the Vulture Peak in Ceylon and in many other places of the Indian subcontinent, Yuthok studied traditional medicine and Buddhist philosophies in depth.

When he was twenty-one, he returned to Tibet and set out to work, dedicating all his effort to working in a clinic and to teaching medicine to his students. Just ten years later, at the age of thirty-one, he had a dream and in a state of clarity, the goddess Dutsima advised him to return to India as it would be of great importance for his future work. He followed the advice and journeyed to India again. He returned to visit the wisdom Dakini Manarava who continued to tutor him, transmitting the Seventy Five Tantras connected to the Eight Branches of Healing. In particular, he received an exceptionally profound teaching on the tantric way to realization which was like the heartblood of the Dakinis and a prophetic indication concerning the propagation of that teaching. This special teaching later came to be known as the Yuthok Nyingthig, The Innermost Essence of Yuthok.

Returning to work in Tibet, he became a doctor and master without equal and was celebrated as Yuthok Yonten Gonpo, meaning Yuthok 'Lord of All Qualities'. He composed The Essence of the Extended and Brief Eight Branches of Healing, the treatise on the Examination of the Pulse, the Three Manuscripts on Medicine, the Small Tantra, the Medical Experience for Students, the Two Commentaries on the Four Medical Tantras, and the Eighteen Supplements to the Four Tantras. He transmitted all his teachings and writings in their entirety to Sumtöng Yeshé Zung but his accomplished disciples were numerous, almost three hundred.

One day, Yuthok was invited by the Governor of Western Tibet to visit the region. Yuthok accepted the invitation and during his stay in Western Tibet, he taught medicine for four months including the Middle Way of Buddhist Philosophy and the Dzogchen or Self-Perfection system. He gave a series of empowerments including the Medicine

Buddha, the Peaceful and Wrathful Deities, Hevajra, Vajra Kilaya, the Guardian of Medicine and the Sages of Medicine. Those who participated in these teachings and empowerments perceived Yuthok in different forms, some saw him as a yogi, some as a sage, some as a great scholar, some people observed him in the midst of rainbows, smelt fragrant perfumes and heard music.

Suddenly one day, fresh Arura fruits all golden in colour fell for an hour within the walls of the Governor's residence and the people rushed to gather the fruit, arguing amongst themselves. Yuthok announced to them that if they had not disturbed the Goddess of Medicine with their greed, the rain would have brought other special medicines.

When his main disciple Sumtöng Yeshé Zung asked Yuthok about the meaning of such special signs, Yuthok explained that the signs had three levels of meanings; an outer, an inner and a secret meaning. In an external or outer level, it indicated that there was no one in Tibet or India who could match Yuthok's knowledge. In an inner sense, it showed that Yuthok had attained the eight great powers (e.g. fast walking) and in a secret sense, it indicated that Yuthok was one and the same with the infinite mandalas of all Buddhas. In particular these were signs that he was an emanation of the doctor of the Buddha, of Padmasambhava, Ashvagosha, Padampa Sangye, Virupa, the famous doctor Kyebu Mela and in Tibet, of Srongtsen Gampo, Yuthok the elder and Gampopa.

Throughout all his life, Yuthok selflessly dedicated himself to others not only by teaching but also donating the medicines he prepared to the sick and giving clothes to the needy.

Once, when Yuthok went to pay homage to a self-originated statue of Buddha, from the heart of the statue emanated light resounding with the mantra of the medicine Buddha and spread everywhere. When the light dissolved, it entered into the head of Yuthok. He remained a while, absorbed with his gaze lost in contemplation and then called upon his student Sumtöng Yeshé Zung Yuthok told him, "You've been with me for twelve years. Now, if you have any doubts that have not been resolved please tell me now, I may soon depart for another land." Sumtöng was shocked and cried at the thought of his master passing away. "You don't need to cry, I will live for sometime more. I told you this just to make you aware of the transitory nature of life". Sumtöng paid homage to the master and made a symbolic offering of the universe, then asked him for the ultimate teaching that would enable him to become a Buddha. In answer, Yuthok taught the Guru Yoga contained in the Yuthok Nyingthig.

When he reached the age of seventysix, Yuthok summoned all his disciples to offer a teaching and presented them with many gifts. On that occasion, he briefly recounted his life story in the following song:

Hey! Listen fortunate ones!
Listen well, people of the world
In particular, you who are gathered here
Even though you have listened much before
All those were meaningless illusory words
Today you will listen to what is really meaningful
Even though you have seen much before
They were just designs of false & deceptive visions.

Today, that which you see will purify the two obscurations
If you do not know who I am
I am the emissary of all Buddhas
I am the refuge of all beings
All the animate and inanimate world
Is pervaded by my body, voice and mind.

The illusory form of this body
Is of the nature of a host of sacred deities
Its materiality is intrinsically pure
And like a rainbow it cannot be grasped, yet
Like the moon's reflection on the water, it appears
everywhere.

The empty sound of my voice is the song of the echo
Reverberating with the sound of the eighty-four thousand
Dharmas
It manifests as a rain of teaching for those who need to
be guided
And sets all beings on the path that ripens and liberates.

In the clarity and emptiness of my mind, the ineffable
authentic state
Bliss is omni pervasive, arising unceasingly and
Emptiness and compassion are undifferentiated
Hence, the phenomena created by mind are naturally
liberated.

Through the shortest instant of time
In an instant I am a fully awakened Buddha
In an instant I travel to hundreds of Buddha fields
In an instant I encounter hundreds of Buddhas
In an instant I manifest hundreds of emanations
In an instant I guide hundreds of beings

And I accomplish the totalities and masteries.

With a faith that does not know uncertainties
Pray without having any doubt!
Even though the cataract of impure vision
Prevents you from seeing all these qualities of mine
In the ordinary perception shared by everyone
I am the doctor who, with the medicine of skilful
compassion
Cures the inner mental illness of the three emotions
The outer illness of the three humours, Wind, Bile and
Phlegm
The title 'doctor' applies to me.

I explain the Buddhist canon and its commentaries by
heart
With logic I overcome the challenges of fundamentalists
I issue the banner of victory of the Buddhist doctrine
The title 'scholar' applies to me.

I went to Sri Parvata and
Robbers created obstacles on my way
But with a gaze I paralysed them all
The title 'siddha' applies to me.

On my way to Odiyana, flesh eating dakinis
Sent meteorites and lightning to strike me
I made the threatening gesture and all the dakinis
collapsed
The title 'siddha' applies to me.

On my way to Ceylon
The boat fell apart in the midst of the waves
I flew like a bird and also saved my companions
The title 'siddha' applies to me.

When I went to the Kali forest
The vapour of venomous snakes spread like dark fog
I meditated on compassion and the fog quickly vanished
The title 'siddha' applies to me.

When I went to Persia
I encountered the army of the Mongols

So I penetrated the rocky mountains back and forth
The title 'siddha' applies to me.

When I visited Swayambhu
I competed with the Bonpos in magic
For half a day I remained sitting in space
The title 'siddha' applies to me.

I went from Bodhgaya to Tibet
Taking only a single day
Carrying a fresh flower as gift
The title 'siddha' applies to me.

At the place of Tshongdu Kormoru in Western Tibet
I prevented the sun from setting and
Caused a rain of Aruras, golden in colour, to fall
The title 'siddha' applies to me.

It would be endless to recount all the events of my life
For one who has gained mind freedom
There are no disturbances caused by earth
Water, fire and wind, gods and demons etc
And by animate and inanimate enemies
He flies in the sky swifter than birds
He dives in the waters with nothing to stop him
He penetrates mountains like a meteorite or lightning
In the midst of fire he is the fire god.

The beings of the degenerate age are of little merit
And few are those who meet and listen to me
Those who see, listen, think, touch me and have faith in
me
Create the sprout of the spirit of enlightenment
Purify negativities accumulated throughout eons
Overcome obstacles and adverse condition of this life
Liberate themselves, liberate others and liberate both
And liberate all their followers.

I will connect to happiness even
Those who, harbouring negative views, harm me
Hence, I will lead them from happiness to happiness
There is no doubt about this.

If you give up your heart and mind to me
Beseech me in a sincere way
Overcome your lack of faith and
Hope in me as a refuge throughout your life
Immediately your two obscurations will diminish
Upon meeting me in reality, in vision or in dream
I will reveal the path to the temporal and ultimate goal.

All of you present now and the students to come
My sons, and disciples remember this!
For the time being, my work of training beings in this
world is complete
I will now go to the pure land of the Medicine Buddha.

Yuthok then proceeded to offer much advice to his student doctors. Thereafter, great light came from the sky intertwined with a net of rainbows, filling the entire sky. That radiance touched his body and, floating into the sky, he departed to the pure land of the Medicine Buddha without leaving any mortal remains.

Yuthok's Disciple Lineage

If every disciple of this great being were counted, they would equal the number of stars in the sky or specks of dust on the earth. His most well known disciples however were Jangmen Lebsé, Belmen Nyima Pel, Jé Yeshé Sung, Tönpa Atsé, Shakrampa Nyima Pel, Yuthok Bumseng and Yuthok Söseng, Sumtöng Yeshé Zung, and Geshé Rokchung.

Among these disciples, Sumtöng Yeshé Zung worked unceasingly for the welfare of others through the manifested play of the seven lotus holding conquerors, and he is counted in the garland of births of my lama the Great Fifth. He was born the son of Rutsam from Darsumpa in Nyemo. He trained in other sciences until he perfected them and then one day, he heard the life story of master Yuthok. His mind was captivated. He decided to seek out teachings in medicine and for twelve years, lived in the service of the master. The Four Tantras: the Essence of Ambrosia Secret Instruction Tantra, a king among tantras due to its profound nature, was at that time expounded only to Yeshé Zung. This clearly indicated that he was truly the main heart disciple of master Yuthok. In his 'Sunlight of Compassion Clearing the Darkness of Suffering' he says:

"In the presence of the great Yuthok, whose name is hard to say, whose nature is the very gnosis, inseparable from every deed, quality, body, speech and mind of every Buddha of every direction and of every time. Through the kindness of the compassion of this great being I, the physician Sumtöng Yeshé Zung born of Rutsam, served him and delighted him with the three ways of pleasing, through devotion in action, speech and thought for many years. Because of this I received the profound essence of the scriptures and instructions, the transmissions and practices in their entirety in the manner of a full vase being poured into another and like a son receiving his inheritance from his father. Every profound and essential point was taught without error and all arose from the churning stick of guidance through experience. I was appointed as his main heart disciple. I can state, not with mere words but from my heart, that this unparalleled and venerable guru is truly the great arhat Vajradhara. Through his blessings I too without difficulty have developed the unmistaken, profound and subtle view, exactly as it is, of that special state of emptiness and compassion combined, thus all auspicious conditions necessary to effortlessly fulfil the needs of oneself and others are in place. In particular, the transmission of the Four Tantras, the very king of all medical scripture, and all the auxiliary texts, has been entrusted to no one else but me. As for the extent of my future lineage, the master delightedly prophesised "Having taken the firm ground of working for living beings until samsara has been emptied, you will be of inconceivable and indescribable help to others through the science of healing."

In his Effortless Accomplishment of the Five Bodies he wrote:

> A person such as I, Jñanadhara
> Son of Rutsam Sumpa
> Heard of the fame of my master from afar
> And just to hear his name gave me joy.
>
> Enduring the journey's hardships I came into his presence
> And by merely seeing his face received his blessings
> Although I had no wealth with which to offer
> I exchanged land for horses and made offerings.
>
> Although I could not serve him physically
> Whatever he commanded I never disobeyed
> Although my practice of the texts was not great
> I studied for three years without distraction.
>
> While staying in Gyaché Nyendrong
> Though I had not ascertained the fundamentals of the teachings
> I made a single prayer and by his great compassion
> He gave me this tantra on the science of healing

He made the pledge without omission, without excess.
Granted the blessings of the Rishi lineage, and said

"So that the one-to-one transmission remains unbroken
Now I am entrusting it to you
For the time being, do not expound it
But keep it as a secret hidden treasure
And unseen by your companions
Write it down secretly as a manuscript
Keep it secret for a whole year
The power of which will bring you siddhi."

As he commanded, so I followed
Sometimes I wrote in secret on mountaintops
Sometimes in the deepest valleys
Sometimes in the deepest forests.

Thirteen years later in the jina horse year
In the Pelkhor temple of Yeru
I put the writing into print
A scripture never before, seen heard or experienced
Now shines like the sun in the sky
May it shine in glory for all living beings.

The master Yuthok Gönpo is like Vidyajñana
And I feel as if I am truly Manasija
I think that surely he was my lama in lives gone by
His kindness was immense and I never forget
To place him upon my head
Grant me constantly your blessings.

This master had so many disciples
But in the early part of his life
Jangmen Pelé of Tsida was the most renowned
Toward the master he was very competitive
And did not penetrate to the root of these teachings
These days what has his fame accomplished?

In the middle part of his life
Khampa Tönpa Atsé was the most renowned
Constantly collating and comparing
Root texts and commentaries of the eight branches
He did not penetrate to the root of these teachings

These days what has his explaining of texts
accomplished?

In the latter part of his life
Geshé Rokchung of the west was the most renowned
He was constantly attached to his family line
And did not penetrate to the root of these teachings
These days who will care for him?

At all times the two sons and two son-in-laws
Carried over familiarity in master-disciple relationship
And did not penetrate to the root of these teachings
These days who looks after the son disciples?

Of the disciples that came from afar
Some only learned one important thing
Some valued the unworthy
Some concentrated only on investigation
Some wrote down whatever came to them
Others returned empty handed
Some saw the practices and then left
Some spent their time singing and dancing
Some just wasted their time
Not penetrating to the root of these teachings
These days how will they heal the sick?

The one who truly gained the teachings
Of the master Yuthok Gönpo was me alone
The stream of his words flowed into me
And if even Kumāra Jīvaka himself were here
I think I would have nothing to ask of him.

I do not need fame and fortune
I have truly met the guru Rishi
There is no way I can be deficient in the teachings.

The heart disciple of Yuthok Yönten Gönpo, master of manifesting and
withdrawing an ocean of mandalas, was Sumtöng Yeshé Zung. As an
author, he composed various works such as the life story of Yuthok
known as 'Effortless Accomplishment of the Five Bodies' or 'Sealed
Biography of Yuthok, Secret Biography', the 'Illuminating Beacon Small
Commentary Collection', the 'Commentary on the Explanatory Tantra'
and the'Treatment of Kangbam - Notes from the Whispered Tradition'.

Mainly, he concentrated on spreading the teachings of the glorious Four Tantras (*rGyud-bZhi*).

Sumtöng's main disciple was Shönu Yeshé and in the Effortless Accomplishment of the Five Bodies it says:

> Vidyajñana was Yuthok Gönpo,
> Manasija was the divine master,
> I am Tsojé Shönu Yeshé.
> He was my master in births without beginning,
> I have been held by the compassion of the lama,
> How kind the lama to this worthy vessel!

The Supreme Doctor Zurkhar Nyamnyid Dorje (1439—1475)

He learnt Tibetan medicine and Buddhism from many great masters such as Rigzin Dorje and Shara Rabjampa. At a very young age, he was a great doctor and helped many suffering patients. It was at the age of sixteen that he had visions of Yuthok in which Yuthok asked him to re-check and re-edit the Four Medical Tantra and the Yuthok Nyingthig as some practitioners were not practicing in the correct way and the teachings needed to be clarified. For the medical part of the Yuthok Nyingthig commentary, he wrote the famous text 'Billions of Instructions on Medicine Relics (*man ngak che wa ring sel*) and contributed substantially to the development of Tibetan medicine and the Yuthok Nyingthig practice.

He realised a great state of emptiness and compassion through Yuthok's teachings and entered into the dimension of the Medicine Buddha.

The Most Outstanding Doctor of Traditional Tibetan Medicine of the 20th Century. A brief biography of Professor Dr Toru Tsenam (1926—2004)

Dr Toru was born in 1926 in Joda County, eastern Tibet. From the age of five, he began studying Tibetan language spoken and written, with his uncle Atse Palden. At the age of twelve, he studied Traditional Tibetan Medicine (TTM) with Lama Guru including the aspects of pulse reading and urine analysis.

From ages fifteen to eighteen, he travelled from Kham on pilgrimage to Lhasa, Bhutan, Nepal and India. When he returned, Kathok Khanpo Legshad Jordan suggested he go to Kathok monastery to learn and further deepen his knowledge of Traditional studies. At Kathok he studied Buddhist philosophy, tantric studies and sutra. He studied and focused on Tibetan medicine with Doctor Tachung Lama Tsering Chophel. It was there he also learned his specialist pharmacopeia skills.

In 1956, he was invited by Toru monastery to teach and there he practice Buddhism and TTM. The monastery bestowed on him the title of Khanchen, the highest position of master at their monastery. High scholars from all over Tibet respected him as a most outstanding Tibetan medicine scholar and doctor. While he was teaching and treating patients at the Toru monastery, he was taken and imprisoned by the Chinese for many years. In fact during the Chinese Cultural Revolution, he spent most of his time in prison, yet even in those terrible conditions, he worked as doctor for the other prisoners and military personnel.

It was 1977 before he was allowed to practice again as a normal doctor in the local village Powo. Here, for the first time since the Chinese Cultural Revolution, he was able to transmit the lineage of making precious pills to about two hundred people. Only through his commitment and abilities was this ancient method of Tibetan medicine preserved.

Not long after that, the Lhasa Mentsee Khang invited him to edit the Tibetan medicine collection book and from there, he went on to teach TTM, the Yuthok Nyingthig, Astrology, Sanskrit and much more. In 1983 the Director of Mentsee Khang invited him to teach Tibetan medicine and Sanskrit. In 1984, he taught Sanskrit and Medicine to the Tibetan medicine teachers. Then in 1987, the Panchen Lama invited him to Beijing's Tibetan Buddhism College to teach Buddhism and the Kagyu tradition. While there, he wrote a few books about the history and philosophy of Buddhism.

He became the vice president of Tibetan medicine collage in Lhasa, Tibet in 1989. He taught the doctors and students from Central Tibet, Qing hai, Gansu, Suchuan, Yun nan, Xingjian and inner Mongolia. In 1990 he taught Sanskrit, and in 1994 he travelled to England and taught TTM at Samye Ling monastery. It was in Chengdu in 1997 that he gave all his personal teachings to many students.

In all, he wrote about fifteen volumes of teachings and works especially on TTM, and his great commentary on the *rGyud-bZhi*. He revealed about 260 types of Tibetan medicinal formulas and saved the pure lineage of Tibetan medicine within the spiritual aspect. His works on Tibetan medicine are:

- The great commentary on the Four Medical Tantra
- An article of the origin of the *rGyud-bZhi*
- An article on TTM and it's pharmacology and sciences
- The relationship between TTM and astrology
- TTM's past and present, and other many articles on TTM

In 2004, he passed way with great signs of liberation from samsara, and he surely departed to the pure land of the Medicine Buddha.

Appendix 3 - The Ngakpa History

The two Yuthoks, the Elder and Younger, were great Ngakpa or Tibetan Yogis. In western society, there is very little information about the great Ngakpa tradition. The following is a brief history of the Tibetan Ngakpa tradition and its masters in the Amdo region of Tibet.

The Ngakpa is the cultural and non-monastic spiritual tradition of the Tibetan people. Padmasambava (*Guru Rinpoche*) is its founder who developed it in the eighth century so that lay people could receive spiritual and cultural education. The Tibetan king Trisong Detsan not only made large contributions to the development of the Ngakpa tradition but as an example to his people, he became a Ngakpa himself.

Ngak Mang (a large group of Ngakpa) was commonly called *Gokar Chanlo De*, which literally means 'The community with white dress and long hair' or more simply, 'The group of White Sangha'. The first group of Ngakpa was called *Je Bang Nyirnya*, and they were twentyfive highly trained disciples of Padmasambava.

The first Ngakpa College was a branch of Samnye Monastery and was called the Ngakpa 'Dud dul Ling'. Students were trained in numerous subjects including Language, Literature, Translation, Agriculture, Medicine, Astrology, Meteorology and Vajrayana studies and practices.

The Ngakpa culture continued to develop and spread all over Central Tibet forming significant principal groups; thirty Sheldrak Ngakpa groups, one hundred and eight Chuon Ngakpa groups and eighty Drag-Yir-Pa Ngakpa groups. Many Ngakpa became highly educated people and practitioners, demonstrating their great abilities. A good example of this is the founder of TTM, Yuthok Yonten Gonpo who was an exceptionally skilled Ngakpa, as were many of his lineage physicians.

In the nineth Century, Tri Ralpa Chan, the third Tibetan Dharma King, became involved in the Ngakpa Tradition and through his dedication and support, the Ngakpa culture florished all over Tibet. The last Tibetan king Lhang Tharma tried his best to eradicate the Buddhist tradition in Tibet but he was not able to destroy the Ngakpa tradition. It is fundamental to native Tibetans. Free from any sectarian beliefs, the Ngakpa tradition continues today in China, Bhutan, Nepal, India and Mongolia, and more recently in the west, with men and women studying and practicing throughout their daily lives.

Yuthok Yonten Gonpo the Younger (1126—1202)

Yuthok the younger is known as the Father of Traditional Tibetan Medicine and of the Yuthok Nyingthig.

Yeshe Tsogyal (777—837)

Tibetan women are recognised as significant contributors to the Ngak Mang. Ngakma (female Ngakpa) such as Yeshe Tsogyal, Machin Labdron and Chusep Jetsun were highly respected practitioners and an inspiration to many Tibetan women. The first Tibetan Ngakma was Yeshe Tsogyal and, as she uncovered many mantras and therapies relating to Tibetan medicine, she is also considered the first female Tibetan doctor.

The Ngakpa Lineage

In the 10th century, a famous Ngakpa named Lhalung Paldor travelled to Amdo and introduced the Vajra seed of the Ngakpa tradition in Rebkong, Tibet. He was particularly skilled in the practices of *Lodorje Drag, Namong* and *Tongtso.*

The descendants of Lhalung Paldor, known as the Eight Great Ngakpa of Rebkong, practiced in eight different places and all of them successfully completed their practices and achieved realisation. Those eight places of retreat are referred to as the Eight Accomplished Places of Retreat. The disciples of the Eight Great Ngakpa continued their ancient and secret spiritual knowledge, integrating it into their daily life.

Adron Khetsun Gyatso (1604—1679)

He was a highly qualified Ngakpa Master who founded one of the earliest Ngakpa houses in Rebkong known as *Adron Nangchen.*

Rigzin Palden Tashi (1688—1743)

He was born into the *rLang* family - one of the four important Tibetan families of that time. He was trained in both the Nyingma and Gelug Buddhist schools.

In his twenties, he travelled to central Tibet where he studied Nyingma practice. After completing his spiritual education and practice in Mendro Ling and Kham Srinmozong, he returned to Rebkong and became a great ambassador for the Ngakpa tradition. During 1727—1742, he travelled to various places, offering teachings to many lay people. Eventually, he formed the Great Group of Rebkong Ngakpa, known as Rebkong Ngak Mang. Through his dedication, thousands of Ngakpa and Ngakma came to Amdo to settle, building many homes. His followers referred to him as the King of the Ngakpa tradition.

Chögyal Ngawang Dargye (1740—1807)

He was a Mongolian king from the Tseshung area in Amdo, and was a highly accomplished scholar, well versed in languages, literature, medicine and astrology. Fulfilling the ancient prophecy of Padmasambhava, he studied the practice of *Kunsang Tapak Tersar.* He successfully completed all practices and also wrote commentaries on them. He trained great Ngakpa such as Shabkar Tsokdrug Rangdrol and Padma Rangdrol. His wife, Rigzin Wangmo, was a Rebkong Ngakma.

Changlung Pelchen Namkha Jigmed (1757—1821)

He was one of the head of the Rebkong Ngak Mang and during his time, the Rebkong Ngak Mang split into two regional groups; a Southern group called *Nyinta* Ngak Mang and a Northern group called *Sribta* Ngak Mang. He founded the Kyung Gon Ngakpa House which was the main place of practice for the Northern group, whose origin is the tradition of *Min-Ling* and *Nyid-rag gter-ma*.

At his initiation of the Eight Herukas, one thousand nine hundred Ngakpa attended the event and in celebration, he offered each of them a *phur-ba* (dagger) as a symbol of the Ngakpa and they became known as the 'Rebkong Ngak Mang 1900 Phur-ba Holders'.

Megsar Kunsang Tubdan Wang Po (1781—1832)

A specialist in Vajrayana studies particularly Vajrakilaya Tantra, he authored a large volume of books about Vajrakilaya Tantra. He also founded Padma Namdrol Ling, a very important Ngakpa House in the Rebkong region.

Shabkha Tsogdruk Rangdrol (1781—1851)

He was a well known Rebkong Ngakpa who founded Tashi Kyil Ngakpa House and wrote twentytwo volumes, which included his Autobiography, Spiritual Songs and Vajrayana philosophy and practices. His written work is well known outside of Tibet and in fact several texts have been translated into many languages including English.

Dzogchen Choying Tobdan Dorje (1785—1848)

He was a brilliant Vajrayana master who founded the 'Dzogchen Namgyal Ling Ngakpa House'. He wrote The Treasure of Sutra and Tantra which contains The Ten Tibetan Studies which has become the main text studied by Ngakpa.

Khamla Tragthug Namkha Gyatso (1788—1851)

Born in Kham, he was an extraordinary Ngakpa master and *Terton* (revealer of hidden treasures). He became head of the Southern Ngakpa and founded Gonlakha Ngakpa House, the main place of practice for the Southern Ngakpa region. The special lineage practices offered at Gonlakha Ngakpa House were the traditions of Longchen Nyingthig and Khamla Tesar.

Terton Natsok Rangdrol (1796—1861)

He revealed many *gter-mas* (hidden treasures) of Dzogchen practices and wrote six volumes of commentaries and explanations about

Vajrayana. He founded Terton Chögar Ngakpa House.

Nyankyi Nangzad Dorje (1798—1874)

One of the main disciples of Shabkar Tsokdrug Rangdrol, he collected and completed Shabkar's work and founded a library of Ngakpa texts.

Alak Jamyang Jigmed Khedrub Gyatso (1929—to date)

Alak Jampyang was born in 1929 in Rebkong, Amdo. At the age of seven, he studied with the Ngakpa Master Jidme Yeshe Nyingpo. He studied philosophy and learned the practice of Buddha Dharma; as part of his practice he did 100 days of yoga training, 100 days of Bardo training, and 100 days of Dzogchen practice.

At the age of twentyone he took up studies in Tibetan medicine and worked as a local doctor helping many people. Between the ages of thirty to forty, he was imprisoned in a Chinese prison and while in prison, he continued to treat & cure many sick people. Many highly qualified masters were also in prison and so Alak Jamyang was able to continue his study and practices, both in Medicine and Dharma. In 1969, he was released from prison and returned home where he worked as a local doctor at Tsekok Tibetan Medicine Hospital.

He received many secret teachings on Tibetan medicine from Trulshig Gyepa Rinpoche and Gedun Tenzin. In the 1980's, he travelled to Lhasa where he received more teachings on Tibetan medicine and importantly, he received the whole teachings of the Yuthok Nyingthig from Khenpo Troru Tsenam. Returning to Amdo, he completed the practice of Yuthok Nyingthig.

For many years he worked tirelessly offering teachings on Medicine and Dharma, treating patients while still managing to continue writing many texts on Medicine. In the year 2000, he was invited by the Larung Centre to visit the Kham areas where he gave intensive teachings on the Yuthok Nyingthig practice and many other teachings. Today he is the main lineage holder of the Yuthok Nyingthig in Amdo, and one of most outstanding Ngakpa Masters.

The Ngakpa lineage continues today and there are many Ngakpa Masters, recognised reincarnations, scholars and great practitioners who continue this ancient tradition. In Amdo, there are approximately 250 Ngakpa Houses and about 6000 practicing Ngakpa including men, women and children.

Appendix 4 - The Yuthok Nyingthig Linage

སངས་རྒྱས་སྨན་བླ།
Medicine Buddha

གུ་རུ་པདྨ་འབྱུང་གནས།
Padmasambava

གཡུ་ཐོག་ཡོན་ཏན་མགོན་པོ།
Yuthok Yonten Gonpo, the Elder

མཁའ་འགྲོ་མ་དཔལ་ལྡན་ཕྲེང་བ།
Dakini Palden Tringva

གཡུ་ཐོག་གསར་མ་ཡོན་ཏན་མགོན་པོ།
Yuthok Yonten Gonpo, the Younger (1126—1201)

སུམ་སྟོན་ཡེ་ཤེས་གཟུངས།
Sumtomg Yeshe Zung (12th century)

གཙོ་བཟེད་གཞོན་ནུ་ཡེ་ཤེས།
Tsozed Shonnu yeshe (12th—13th century)

སངས་རྒྱས་ཡེ་ཤེས།
Zangton Sangye Yeshe

རིན་ཆེན་རྡོ་རྗེ།
Khetsun Rinchen Dorje

བྲང་ཏི་དངོས་གྲུབ་རྒྱ་མཚོ།
Tranti Mangtho Ngodrub Gyatso

བྲང་ཏི་དཀོན་མཆོག་རྒྱལ་མཚན།
Tranti Konchog kyab

བྲང་ཏི་དཀོན་མཆོག་སྐྱབས།
Tranti Konchog Kyab (14th century)

ཟུལ་ཕུ་རིག་འཛིན་སྨན་མོ་རིན་ཆེན།
Zulphu Rigzin Manmo Rinchen

རྣལ་འབྱོར་བསོད་ནམས་དབང་པོ།
Naljor Sodnam Wangpo

རྣལ་འབྱོར་ཆེན་པོ།
Naljor Chenpo

རི་ཁྲོད་ཞིག་པོ།
Ritrod Shigpo

ཟུར་མཁར་མཉམ་ཉིད་རྡོ་རྗེ།
Zurkhar Nyamnyid Dorje (1439—1475)

དཔག་དབོན་དཀོན་མཆོག་བཟང་པོ།
Trakbon Konchog Sangpo

དཀོན་མཆོག་ནམ་མཁའ་རིན་ཆེན།
Kongchen Namkha Rinchen Pel

ལེགས་ལྡན་རྡོ་རྗེ།
Legdan Dorje

བཀྲ་ཤིས་སྟོབས་རྒྱལ།
Tashi Tobgya

བྱང་བདག་རིག་འཛིན་ངག་དབང་།
Changdag Rigzin Ngagwang

ཟུར་ཆེན་ཆོས་དབྱིངས་རང་གྲོལ།
Zurchen Choying Rangdrol

ངག་དབང་བློ་བཟང་རྒྱ་མཚོ།
Ngakwang Lobsan Gyatso

བློ་བཟང་ཚེ་དབང་།
Losang Tsewang

ཀུན་བཟང་གྲོལ་མཆོག
KunSang Drolchog

ཆོས་འབྱོར་རྒྱལ་མཚོ།
Chojor Gyatso

རིག་འཛིན་བཟང་པོ།
Rigzin Sangpo

པདྨ་གསང་སྔགས་བསྟན་འཛིན།
Padma Sangngak Tenzin

ཆོས་ཀྱི་རྒྱལ་མཚན།
Chokyi Gyaltsen

མཐུ་སྟོབས་རྣམ་རྒྱལ།
Thutob Namgyal

བསྟན་འཛིན་མཐུ་སྟོབས།
Tenzin Thutob

བྱམས་པ་བསྟན་འཕེལ།
Champa Tenpel

ཆོས་ཀྱི་སེང་གེ།
Chokyi Senge

རྟ་ཆུང་བླ་མ།
Tachung Lama

མཁན་ཆེན་ཁྲོ་རུ་ཚེ་རྣམ།
Khanchen Troru Tsenam

མཁན་པོ་ཚུལ་ཁྲིམས་རྒྱལ་མཚན།
Khanpo Tsultrin Gyaltsen

མཁས་གྲུབ་མི་བསྐྱོད་ཆོང་།
Kyedrub Michod (1929)

Appendix 5 - Yuthok Nyingthig Ngöndro, Mantras & Prayers

Prayer to Yuthok - The One of Secret Form
(*Gangku Sang-chen-ma*)

གང་སྐུ་གསང་ཆེན་མ།

ན་མོ་གུ་རུ།
Na mo guru
Homage to the Guru

གང་གི་སྐུ་ཡི་གསང་ཆེན་མཆོག །
Gang gi ku yi sang chen chog
Whose supreme secret body

དངོས་པོ་ཀུན་ཁྱབ་བདེ་བ་ཆེ། །
Ngö po kun kyab de wa che
Is the nature of Great Bliss that pervades all existence

རྣམ་ཀུན་མཆོག་ལྡན་རྡོ་རྗེའི་དབྱིངས། །
Nam kün chog den dorje ying
In all ways supremely endowed with the Vajra Realm

མཚུངས་བྲལ་གུ་ནའི་སྐུར་ཕྱག་འཚལ། །
Tsung dral gu nai kur chak tsel
To Yuthoks incomparable form, we prostrate

གང་གི་གསུང་གི་གསང་ཆེན་མཆོག །
Gang gi sung gi sang chen chog
He whose supreme secret speech

ষ্ণ'য়য়য়'য়ৢৢৢৢ৾ড়ৢৢৢৢৢৢৢৢৢৢৢৢ৽৽

Dra drak kün kyab shom drel wa

Is the indestructible quality that pervades all sound

བརྒྱད་ཁྲི་བཞི་སྟོང་ཆོས་སྒྲ་སྒྲོགས།།

Gye tri shi tong chö dra drog

Roaring the sound of the 84,000 dharmas

མཚུངས་བྲལ་གུ་ནའི་གསུངས་ཕྱག་འཚལ།།

Tsung dral gu nei sung chag tsal

To Yuthok's incomparable speech, we prostrate

གང་གི་ཐུགས་ཀྱི་གསང་ཆེན་མཆོག།

Gang gi thüg kyi sang chen chog

He whose supreme secret mind

སྤྲོས་པ་ཀུན་བྲལ་བདེ་བ་ཆེ།།

Trö pa kün drel de wa che

Is unconditioned Great Bliss

ཤེས་རབ་ཕ་རོལ་ཕྱིན་ལ་གནས།།

She rab pha rol chin la ne

Dwelling in the Perfection of Wisdom

མཚུངས་བྲལ་གུ་ནའི་ཐུགས་ཕྱག་འཚལ།།

Tsung drel gu nai thüg chag tsal

To Yuthok's incomparable mind, we prostrate

རྒྱལ་བ་ཀུན་ཀྱང་འདྲེན་པ་ཁྱེད།།

Gyel wa kün kyang dren pa kye

You who are the leader of all the Buddhas entirely

ཁྱེད་ལས་གཞན་པའི་སྐྱོབ་པ་ནི།།

Che le shen pai kyob pa ni
There is no refuge other than you

འགྲོ་བ་ཀུན་ལས་འགང་མ་མཆིས།།

Dro wa kün le gang ma chi
For all sentient beings

དེའི་ཕྱིར་ཁྱེད་ལ་སྐྱབས་སུ་མཆི།།

De chir che la kyab su chi
Because of this, in you I take refuge

བྱིས་པས་ཁྱེད་མཚན་མ་ཐོས་པར།།

Chi pe che tsen ma tö pam
Immature beings who haven't heard your name

ཐོས་ཀྱང་གུས་པར་མི་བསྟེན་པར།།

Tö kyang gü par mi ten par
Or if they are able to hear your name but cannot be taught

དེ་ལས་སྙིང་རྗེ་གཞན་མེད་པས།།

De le nying je shen me pe
For them, there is only compassion

བརྩེ་བའི་ཁྱེད་ཀྱིས་རྗེས་སུ་བཟུང་།།

Tse we kye kyi je su zung
Lead them with your loving kindness

ཁྱེད་ཀྱི་མཚན་ཐོས་སྐྱབས་སོང་བའི།།

Che kyi tsän thö kyab song vei
Through hearing your name and taking refuge in you

དེ་ནི་ནམ་ཡང་སྲིད་མཚོར་མིན།།

De ni nam yang si tsor min

They will no longer be in the ocean of samsara

དེ་ཕྱིར་མིག་ཆུ་གཡོ་བཞིན་དུ།།

De chir mik chu yo shin du

Because of this, with eyes filled with tears

སྙིང་ནས་དུས་ཀུན་གསོལ་བ་འདེབས།།

Nying ni dü kün sol va deb

I pray to you at all times from my heart

རབ་འབྱམས་རྒྱལ་བའི་དཀྱིལ་འཁོར་མཆོག།

Rab jam gyal wai kyil kor chog

Infinite supreme mandalas of the Buddhas

གསང་ཆེན་ཁྱེད་སྐུར་རོ་གཅིག་པས།།

Sang chen che kur ro chig pe

Are 'one taste' to your supreme body

དེ་རིང་ཁོ་ནར་མངོན་སུམ་དུ།།

De ring kho nar ngön sum du

Today, right now and in actuality

མཁའ་ཁྱབ་འགྲོ་བས་ཐོབ་པར་ཤོག།

Kha chab dro we tob par shog

May all sentient beings pervading space attain this

Ati Sarwa mangalam.
May virtue spread.

Written by Sumtöng Yeshé Zung

Refuge Prayer

སྐྱབས་འགྲོ།

Taking Refuge in Yuthok, the Perfect Medicine Guru.

ན་མོ།

Namo

རིགས་འདུས་བདེ་གཤེགས་རྡོ་རྗེ་འཆང་།།

Rig dü de sheg Dorje Chang

You who are the union of all sugatas and Vajrdahara

ཕྱོགས་དུས་དཀོན་མཆོག་གསུམ་གྱི་དངོས།།

Chog dü kön chog sum gi ngö

Essence of the Three jewels in the ten directions and three times

བདག་གཞན་བྱང་ཆུབ་མ་ཐོབ་པར།།

Dak shen chang chub ma tob bar

Until I and all others achieve enlightenment

སྙིང་ནས་ཉེ་བར་སྐྱབས་སུ་མཆི།།

Nying ne nye war kyab su chi

From my inner heart I take refuge in you.

(Repeat 101 times)

Bodhicitta – the practice of compassion

སེམས་བསྐྱེད།

Teg chen gyi mön zuk gi sem kye pa la
The Mahayana Bodhicitta of aspiration and entering

སངས་རྒྱས་ཆོས་དང་ཚོགས་ཀྱི་མཆོག་རྣམས་ལ།།

Sangye chö dang tshog kyi chog nam la
The Buddha, dharma and supreme assembly (sangha)

བྱང་ཆུབ་བར་དུ་བདག་ནི་སྐྱབས་སུ་མཆི།།

Chang chub bar du dag ni kyab su chi
Until enlightenment I take refuge in you

བདག་གིས་སྦྱིན་སོགས་བགྱིས་པའི་བསོད་ནམས་ཀྱིས།།

Dag gi jin sog gyi pai sö nam kyi
I will, through the merit of generosity and so on

འགྲོ་ལ་ཕན་ཕྱིར་སངས་རྒྱས་འགྲུབ་པར་ཤོག།

Dro la pen chir sang gye drub par shog
Achieve Buddhahood for the benefit of all sentient beings.

(Repeat 101 times)

The Four Immeasurables

ཚད་མེད་བཞི།

སེམས་ཅན་ཐམས་ཅད་བདེ་བ་དང་བདེ་བའི་རྒྱུ་དང་ལྡན་པར་གྱུར་ཅིག།

Sem chen tham che de wa dang de wai gyu dang den par gyur chik

May all beings have happiness and the causes of happiness

སེམས་ཅན་ཐམས་ཅད་སྡུག་བསྔལ་དང་སྡུག་བསྔལ་གྱི་རྒྱུ་དང་བྲལ་བར་གྱུར།

Dug ngel dang dug ngel gyi gyu dang dral war gyur chik

May all beings be free from suffering and the causes of suffering

སེམས་ཅན་ཐམས་ཅད་སྡུག་བསྔལ་མེད་པའི་བདེ་བ་དང་མི་བྲལ་བར་གྱུར་ཅིག།

Dug ngel med pai dewa dampa dang min drel war gyur chik

May all beings never be separated from the supreme joy that is beyond all suffering

སེམས་ཅན་ཐམས་ཅད་ཉེ་རིང་ཆགས་སྡང་གཉིས་དང་བྲལ་བའི་བཏང་སྙོམས་ཆེན་པོ་ལ་གནས་པར་གྱུར་ཅིག།

Nye ring chag dang nyi dang dral wei dang nyom chen po la

May all beings abide in equanimity, free from attachment, aversion and sorrow.

(Repeat 3, 7 or 21 times)

Prostration Prayer

བསྟོད་ཕྱག

This is for purification of the body and to accumulate merit.

གང་གི་དྲིན་གྱིས་བདེ་ཆེན་ཉིད།།

Gang gi drin gyi dechen nyi
From the kindness of Great Bliss itself

སྐད་ཅིག་ཉིད་ལ་འཆར་བ་གང་།།

Ke chig nyi la char war gang
Instantly arises inside of us

བླ་མ་རིན་ཆེན་ལྟ་བུའི་སྐུ།།

Lama rinchen ta bui ku
The guru with jewel-like form

རྡོ་རྗེ་འཆང་ཞབས་པད་ལ་འདུད།།

Dorje chen shab pä la dü
I prostrate at the feet of the Vajra Holder.

(Repeat 101 times)

Mandala Offering

For realising inner knowledge and to gather the two accumulations (merit and wisdom)

བདག་གཞན་ལུས་དང་ལོངས་སྤྱོད་དུས་གསུམ་གྱི།།

Dag shen lü dang long chö dü sum gyi

The body, possessions and pleasures of myself and others, of the three times

དགེ་ཚོགས་དང་བཅས་རི་གླིང་ཉི་ཟླ་སོགས།།

Ge tsog dang che ri ling nyi da sog

And all accumulations virtues, together with Mount Meru, the four continents, the sun and moon and so on

ཀུན་བཟང་མཆོད་སྤྲིན་བསམ་ཡས་སྤྲུལ་བྱས་ཏེ།།

Kun zang chö trin sam ye trül jehteh

The emanated inconceivable offering clouds of Kuntuzangpo

བླ་མ་དཀོན་མཆོག་ཐུགས་རྗེ་ཅན་ལ་འབུལ།།

La ma kön chog thük je chen la bül

I offer to the compassionate Lama, the Three Jewels

བསོད་ནམས་ཡེ་ཤེས་ཚོགས་གཉིས་རྫོགས་པར་ཤོག།

Sö nam ye shay tsok nyi dzog par shog

May the two accumulations of merit and wisdom be perfected.

(Repeat 101 times)

Mantra of Circumambulation

བསྐོར་བ།

This is to purify the body's chakras and channels.

In the original text, it states one mandala offering followed by one circumambulation. As this is not practical, do offerings first followed by circumambulations.

Namo da sha daki tira ka la sarva ratna
tra ya ya nama prada cha
su pra dasha. sarva papam bisho dani so ha

Mantra of Medicine Buddha

སངས་རྒྱས་སྨན་བླའི་སྔགས།

Tayata Om
bhe-kha-dze bhe-kha-dze
ma-ha bhe-kha-dze
raza samud-gate so-ha
(Repeat 101 times)

Vajrasattva Mantra

རྡོ་རྗེ་སེམས་དཔའི་བསྒོམ་སྒྲུབ།།

རང་གི་སྤྱི་བོར་པད་ཟླ་བའི་སྟེང་།།
Rang gi chi wor pe dai teng
Above my head in a white lotus moon disc

ཧཱུྃ་དཀར་ལས་གྲུབ་རྡོ་རྗེ་སེམས།།
Hung kar lei drub Dorje Sem
On which a white Hung becomes Vajrasattva

ལོངས་སྤྱོད་རྫོགས་སྐུའི་ཆ་ལུགས་ཅན།།
Long chö dzok kui cha lug chen
In manner and accoutrements of Samboghakaya,

ཕྱག་གཉིས་རྡོ་རྗེ་དྲིལ་བུ་འཛིན།།
Chak nyi dorje drilbu dzin
The two hands holding vajra and bell.

ཐུགས་ཀར་ཟླ་སྟེང་ཧཱུྃ་གི་མཐར།།
Thük kar da ting Hung gi thar
At his heart is a moon disc with the syllable Hung,

ཡི་གེ་བརྒྱ་བའི་སྔགས་ཀྱིས་བསྐོར།།
Yi ge gya pai ngag kyi kor
Surrounded by the hundred syllable mantra

འོད་འཕྲོས་འཕགས་མཆོད་འགྲོ་དོན་བྱས།།
Ö trö phag chö dro dön jeh
Which radiates light which offers to the Buddhas and benefits sentient beings.

བདུད་རྩི་མཐེབ་སོར་ནས་འཛག་པས།།
Dütsi theb sor ne dzag pai
Nectar pours from Vajrasattva's big toe,

རང་གི་ལུས་བགྲུས་སྡིག་སྒྲིབ་ཀུན།།
Rang gi lü tru dig drib kün
Washing through my body; all stains and obscurations

མ་ལུས་བྱང་ཞིང་དག་པར་གྱུར།།
Ma lü chang shing dag par gyur
With exception are completely cleansed and become purified.

The '100 Syllable Purification Mantra'

Om Vajrasattva samaya ma nu palaya
Vajrasattva tenopa tishda dri-dho me bhava
suto-shayo me bhava supo-shayo me bhava
anu-rakto me bhava sarva siddhi me pra-ya-tsa
sarva karma sutsa me tsitam shre-yam kuru-hum
ha ha ha ha ho!
bhagavan sarva tathagata vajra ma-me muntsa
vajra bhava maha samaya sattva
Ah Hung Phat
(Repeat 101 times)

The short mantra

Om banzar sato hung
(Sanskrit, Om vajra sattva hum)

Kusali Body Offering Practice

ཀུ་ས་ལི། ལུས་སྦྱིན།

མདུན་མཁར་བླ་མ་སྨན་པའི་རྒྱལ་པོ་ལ།།

Dün kar lama man pai gyal po la

In the sky in front is the lama, King of Medicine

མགྲོན་རིགས་བཞིས་བསྐོར་སྤྲིན་ཕུང་གཏིབ་ལྟར་བཞུགས།།

Drön rig shi kor trin pung tib tar shuk

Residing amidst the four classes of guests, like a massed gathering of clouds

རང་སེམས་དབྱིངས་ཐོན་རྡོ་རྗེ་རྣལ་འབྱོར་མ།།

Rang sem ying tön Dorje Naljorma

One's own consciousness is ejected into space

དམར་མོ་གྲི་ཐོད་འཛིན་པའི་སྐུ་རུ་གྱུར།།

Mar mo dri tö dzin pai ku ru gyur

Becoming the form of Vajrayogini holding a curved knife and skull cap

བེམ་པོའི་ཐོད་པ་ཕྱག་གཡས་ཀྱི་གུག་གིས།།

Bem poi thö pa chak ye dri gug gi

With her driguk, she cuts open the skull of our corpse

བྲེགས་ཏེ་རང་བྱུང་ཐོད་པའི་སྐྱེད་པུར་བཙུགས།།

Dreg te rang chung thö pai gyed pur tsug

Placing it on a self-arisen hearth of skulls

དེ་ནང་ཤ་རུས་ཏིལ་འབྲུ་ཙམ་དུ་གསིལ།།

De nang sha rü til dru tsam du sil

Inside the skull, the flesh and bones are chopped fine as mustard seeds

ཨེ་རླུང་སྦྱོར་བའི་ཟག་མེད་བདུད་རྩིའི་མཚོ།།

Me lung jor vei sag med düd tsi tso

Through conjoined fire and wind, it becomes an inexhaustible ocean of nectar

ནམ་མཁའི་ཁྱོན་གང་མཆོད་སྤྲིན་ཟད་མི་ཤེས།།

Nam khai kyön gang chö trin ze mi shay

Filling the breadth of space with endless offering clouds

མགྲོན་རིགས་སོ་སོའི་བཞེས་རྒུར་འཆར་བར་གྱུར།།

Drön rig so soi shay gur char var gyur

Whatever is wished for or desired arises for each class of guest

ཐུགས་ལས་མཆོད་པའི་ལྷ་མོ་གྲངས་མེད་སྤྲོས།།

Thuk leh chö pai lhamo drang meh trö

Through countless offering, goddesses emanated from the heart of Vajrayogini

ཨོཾ་ཨཱ་ཧཱུྃ།

Om Ah Hung (Repeat 101 times)

དཀོན་མཆོག་རྩ་གསུམ་སྲིད་ཞིའི་མགྲོན་རྣམས་ལ།།

Kön chog tsa sum si shui drön nam la

The Three Jewels and Three Roots, guests of apparent existence

གུས་པས་འབུལ་ལོ་ཚོགས་གཉིས་རྫོགས་པར་ཤོག།

Gü pei bul lo tsog nyi nyur dzog shog

Offering with devotion to perfect the two accumulations

དཔལ་མགོན་ཆོས་སྐྱོང་ཡོན་ཏན་མགྲོན་རྣམས་ལ།།

Pal gön chö kyong yön ten drön nam la

Glorious dharma protectors, the Guests of Quality

འབུལ་ལོ་ལས་དང་དངོས་གྲུབ་འགྲུབ་པར་མཛོད།།

Bül lo le dang ngö drub drub par dzö
Through offering to you, perform activity and grant siddhi

འགྲོ་བ་རིགས་དྲུག་སྙིང་རྗེའི་མགྲོན་རྣམས་ལ།།

Dro wa rig druk nying jei drön nam la
Beings of the six realms, Guests of Compassion,

སྦྱིན་པས་སྡུག་བསྔལ་ཀུན་ཞི་བདེ་ལྡན་ཤོག།

Jin pe dug ngel kün shi de den shog
Through generosity, may your suffering be pacified and may you have happiness,

རང་སེམས་འཁྲུལ་བའི་སྒྲིབ་པའི་གཞན་དབང་ལས།།

Rang sem trul pai drib pai shen wang le
Our mind, under the power of illusion and obscuration

ཀུན་བཏགས་གཉིས་སུ་སྣང་བའི་ཆོས་རྣམས་ཀུན།།

Kün tak nyi su nang wai chö nam kün
Phenomena are imputed as dualistic appearances

གདོད་ནས་མི་དམིགས་སྤྲོས་བྲལ་ནམ་མཁའ་ལྟར།།

Dö ne mi mig trö dral nam kha tar
Primordially they are non-conceptual and unfabricated like the sky

ཡོངས་གྲུབ་དེ་བཞིན་ཉིད་ཀྱི་དབྱིངས་སུ་ཨ།།

Yong drub de shin nyid kyi ying su Ah
In the sphere of ultimate Suchness - Ah!

Tsog dü (Jigme Lingpa Ganapuja)

Ram Yam Kam

ༀ་ཨ་ཧུ༔།

Om Ah Hung

ཚོགས་རྫས་འདོད་ཡོན་ཡེ་ཤེས་རོལ་པའི་རྒྱན༔།

Tsog dze dö yön ye she rol pe gyen

Tsog substances, the five sense pleasure, ornamented by wisdom,

ཚོགས་རྗེ་ཚོགས་བདག་རིག་འཛིན་བླ་མ་དང་༔།

Tsog je tsog dag rig dzin lama dang

Masters and lords of the tsok, knowledge-holder lamas,

གདན་གསུམ་དཀྱིལ་འཁོར་གནས་ཡུལ་ཉེར་བཞིའི་བདག༔།

Den sum kyil khor ne yül nyer shi dak

Masters of three seats and mandalas, the twenty-four pure realms,

དཔའ་བོ་མཁའ་འགྲོ་དམ་ཅན་ཆོས་སྐྱོང་རྣམས༔།

Pa wo kha dro dam chen chö kyong nam

Dakas and dakinis, samaya-holding protectors,

འདིར་གཤེགས་ལོངས་སྤྱོད་ཚོགས་ཀྱི་མཆོད་པ་བཞེས༔།

Dir sheg long chö tsog kyi chö pa she

Come here and enjoy the offerings of the ganapuja

འགལ་འཁྲུལ་ནོངས་དང་དམ་ཚིག་ཉམས་ཆག་བཤགས༔།

Gal trül nong dang dam tsig nyam chag shag

I confess all confusions, mistakes and broken samaya,

ཕྱི་ནང་བར་ཆད་ཆོས་ཀྱི་དབྱིངས་སུ་གྲོལ༔།

Chi nang bar che chö kyi ying su drol

All outer and inner obstacles are liberated into the Dharma,

ལྷག་གཏོར་བཞེས་ལ་འཕྲིན་ལས་འགྲུབ་པར་མཛོད།།

Lhag tor she la trin le drub par dzö

Please take the remainder torma and perform all activity.

Guru dewa dakini
ganachakra sarva puja
ucha balingta
kha kha khahi kahi

Jigme Lingpa

Dedication Prayer

དགེ་བ་འདི་ཡིས་མྱུར་དུ་བདག །

Ge wa di yi nyur du dag
By the merit, may we quickly

སྨན་རྒྱལ་གཡུ་ཐོག་འགྲུབ་གྱུར་ནས།།

Men gyal Yuthok drub gyur ne
Achieve the state of Yuthok, the King of Medicine

འགྲོ་བ་གཅིག་ཀྱང་མ་ལུས་པ།།

Dro wa chik kyang ma lü pa
And through this, may all beings,

དེ་ཡི་ས་ལ་འགོད་པར་ཤོག །

De yi sa la gö par shog
Be placed on this level.

Mantra of Interdependence

Om ye Dharma
hetu pra-bhawa
he-tun teshun
tathagato haya-wadet
teshun tsa yo niro-dha
ewam wadi
maha sharmana so-ha

GLOSSARY

Expression	Wylie transliteration	Description
Bodhicitta	*Byang sems*	Compassion – the compassionate desire to gain enlightenment for the benefit of all living beings.
Bodhisattva	*jang chub sem pa*	A being pledged to achieve complete enlightenment as a Buddha, in order to benefit all other beings
Gom	*bsGom*	A Tibetan Buddhist method of concentrated meditation
Bhumis	-	Sanskrit term meaning plane, storey or level. Refers to the meditation stages to enlightenment.
Chagtsel	*Phyag 'tshal*	Prostration
Chenrezig	*Spyan ris gzigs*	Buddha of Compassion, known also as Avalokiteshvara
Chegom	*dpyad bsgom*	Analytical meditation. The text 'Wheel of Analytical Meditation' (Tib. Chegom Khorloma; Wyl. dpyad sgom 'khor lo ma) was composed by Mipham Rinpoche in 1891
Five Dhyani Buddhas	*Rgyal rigs lnga*	The Five Buddha Families represent 5 qualities of Buddha
Dzogchen	*rDzogschen*	Great completion meditation
Gyudshi	*rGyud-bZh*	The four medical tantra

Expression	Wylie transliteration	Description
Gyergom	*gyer bsgom*	Chanting meditation
Jamyang	*'jam pai dbyang*	Wisdom Buddha
Karma	*las rgyu 'bras*	Literally means action. The theory of cause and effect
Mahamudra	*Phyag rgya chen po*	(Tib: Chagya Chenpo) The great meditation. It literally means 'great seal' or 'great symbol'.
Mantra	*Sngags*	(Tib: Ngak) Chanting for the protection of mind
Nangtong	*Snangstong*	The union of appearance and emptiness
Ngakpa	*Sngags pa*	Tibetan Yogis
Om Ah Hung	*Om A Hum*	Breathing sound or purification sound
Rainbow body	*'ja lus*	The highest spiritual realisation in the Tibetan spiritual tradition. The dissolution of the physical body into the essence of the 5 elements, disappearing into a 'body of light' typically leaving behind only fragments of hair and finger nails.
Randrol	*rang grol*	Self liberation
Rigpa	*Rigpa*	Awareness
Rishi	*Drangsrong*	Ancient sages
Rtsapra	*Rtsapra*	Pulse divination

Tendrel	*Rten'brel*	Interdependence.
Terma	*gter-ma*	Literally means "treasure" and refers to hidden spiritual teachings
Torma	*Gtorma*	Spiritual cake for offering
Tsogchod	*Tschogs mchod*	Puja practice
Tummo	*Gtummo*	Divine fire yoga
Vajrayana	*Rdo rje theg pa*	The path of Non-dual
Vajrayogini	*Rdorje mal 'byor ma*	Non-dual dakini

Bibliography and References

Yuthok Nyingthig (Tib. gyuthog snying thig)
Original text 2005 NgakMang edition
Beijing National Publishing House, Beijing, China

Gyu Shi, Four Medical Tantra (Tib. gsorig rgyud bzhi)
Tibet National Publishing House, 1982

Yuthok Sarnying Namthar
(Tib. gyu thog gsar rnying gi rnam thar)

Dar mo sman rams pa,
mi rigs dpe skrung khang, 1982, Bejing, China

Words of my Perfect Teacher

Paltrul Rinpoche
Vistaar Publications, India

A Guide to the Words of my Perfect Teacher

Khenpo Ngawang Pelsang
Shambala Boston, London

Ngakmang History

Hungchen Chenagtsang
National Publishing House of Beijing, China 2003

The Author

Dr Nida Chenagtsang was born in Amdo, Tibet. Interested in the traditional medicine of his people, Dr Nida began his early medical training at the local Traditional Tibetan Medicine Hospital. Later he gained scholarship entry to Lhasa Tibetan Medical University and completed his medical training in 1996. Dr Nida obtained his practical training at the Traditional Tibetan Medicine Hospitals in Lhasa (Lhasa Mentsi Khang) and Lhoka.

Dr Nida has published a number of articles and several books on Traditional Tibetan Medicine. He has extensively researched ancient Tibetan medicinal treatments, specialising in the revival of external therapies, which has brought him high acclaim in the field of Tibetan Medicine in both the East and West. Dr Nida is Director of the International Academy for Traditional Tibetan Medicine (IATTM) and the co-founder of the International Ngak Mang Institute (NMI), established to preserve and maintain the Rebkong Ngakpa culture within modern Tibetan society.

Dr Nida's teachings are widely known throughout Asia, Europe, Russia, the USA and Australia, where he has trained students in Traditional Tibetan Medicine, Ku Nye Massage, Mantra Healing, Diet and Behaviour, Dream Analysis, Sa Che (geomancy), as well as Birth and Death according to Tibetan Medicine. All courses, seminars and public talks are organised through the IATTM and NMI.

Fluent in English, Dr Nida is an experienced and knowledgeable communicator with a sophisticated ability to teach the subtleties of these traditional modalities to westerners.

IATTM

The International Academy for Traditional Tibetan Medicine (IATTM) was established in 2006 in order to ensure the integrity and authenticity of Traditional Tibetan Medicine teachings and to promote the continuity of practice of Traditional Tibetan Medicine (TTM).

TTM is a holistic system, meaning that it addresses the individual's needs as a whole – body, mind and spirit – in an integrated way. This includes the individual's internal environment, as well as the way that the individual interacts with the external environment.

It is the sincere aim of the IATTM to keep the spirit of Traditional Tibetan Medicine alive and functioning effectively in the modern world.

Traditional Tibetan Medicine has the capacity to be of great benefit to all in the current economic and social climate.

It is the aim of the International Academy for Traditional Tibetan Medicine to provide courses and training of the highest standard possible, as well as to provide accurate up-to-date information on Traditional Tibetan Medicine as it is currently practised.

IATTM activities include public talks on TTM, specialty courses on TTM, psychology and related healing sciences, facilitation of study tours to Tibet, wellbeing courses and retreats, and publication of the Journal of Traditional Tibetan Medicine - an academic journal of TTM and related topics.

For more information go to iattm.net

CPSIA information can be obtained
at www.ICGtesting.com
Printed in the USA
BVOW05s1128040117
472554BV00010B/150/P